This book belongs to:

____

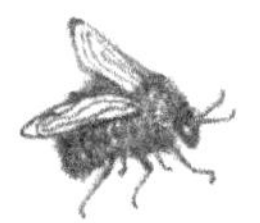
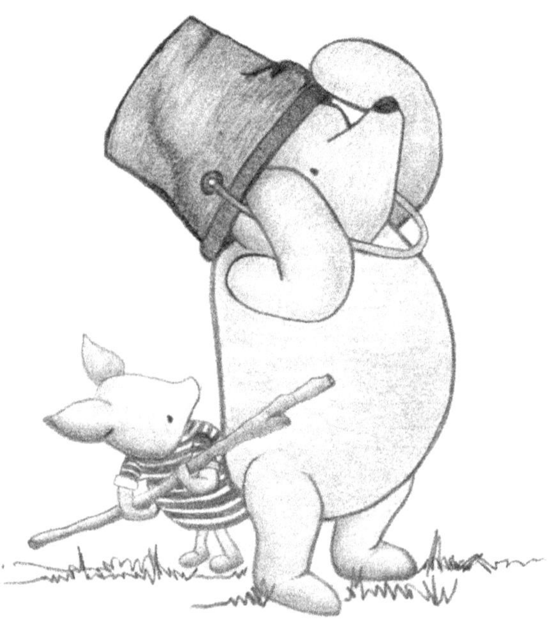

Be Brave

ABCs of Inspiration
for Cancer Patients
from
Winnie the Pooh & Friends

By Carolyn Gundrum

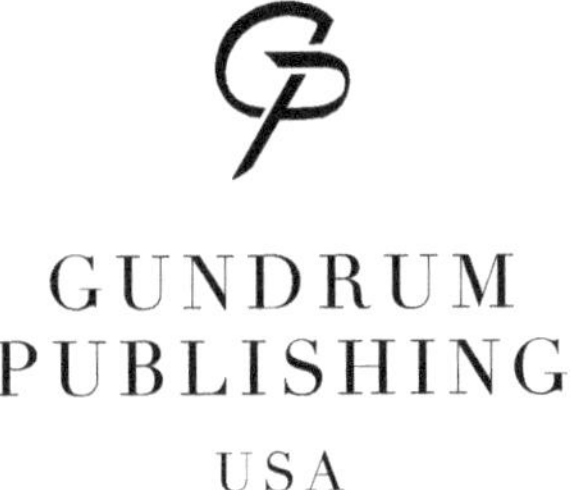

GUNDRUM
PUBLISHING
USA

Book cover by Carolyn Gundrum
Design and layout by Chris Siarkiewicz

First edition 2023
ISBN 979-8-9875260-0-2

For Chris, Stephanie & Sharon

My heart belongs to my family and friends
for helping me beat cancer.

My sister Sharon Murphy was my main driver and advocate
before my son Chris arrived and after he left.

My son Chris flew in for a month from New York to care for me daily
and drive me to and from many appointments. He tried to make me
eat but it was tough going! We did have our heads shaved after my
hair started falling out.

My daughter Stephanie called from Las Vegas daily
to keep on top of my situation.

My neighbors at River Chase are so caring and amazing.
My friends from British Columbia, Michigan, Indiana and Nevada are
so thoughtful and giving. I loved the cards the presents, the toques
and the food!

My Oncologist, Dr. Kristin Thorp, my Radiologist, Dr. Shripal Bhavsar
and their entire staff are wonderful.

A is for Adventure.

"As soon as I saw you, I knew an adventure was going to happen." – Winnie

This is a journey. We can-cer-vive! This may be a scary journey, but be brave. You will learn a lot.

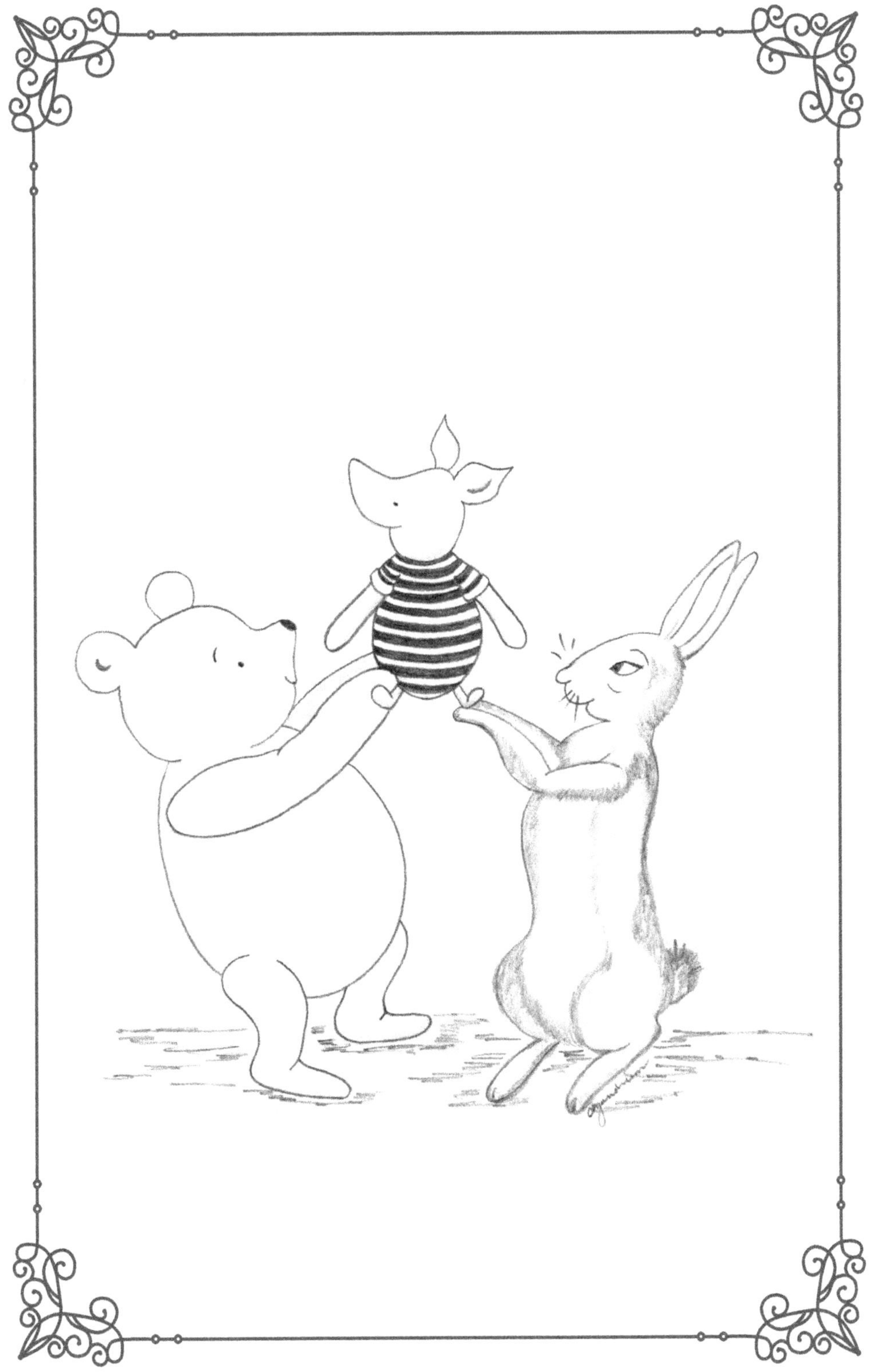

B is for balloon.

"Nobody can be uncheered with a Balloon"
said Pooh.

Have someone order you a brightly colored helium balloon to take with you to chemo or hang on your bed. Name it. Tell it you are a Warrior and you will beat this cancer with style!

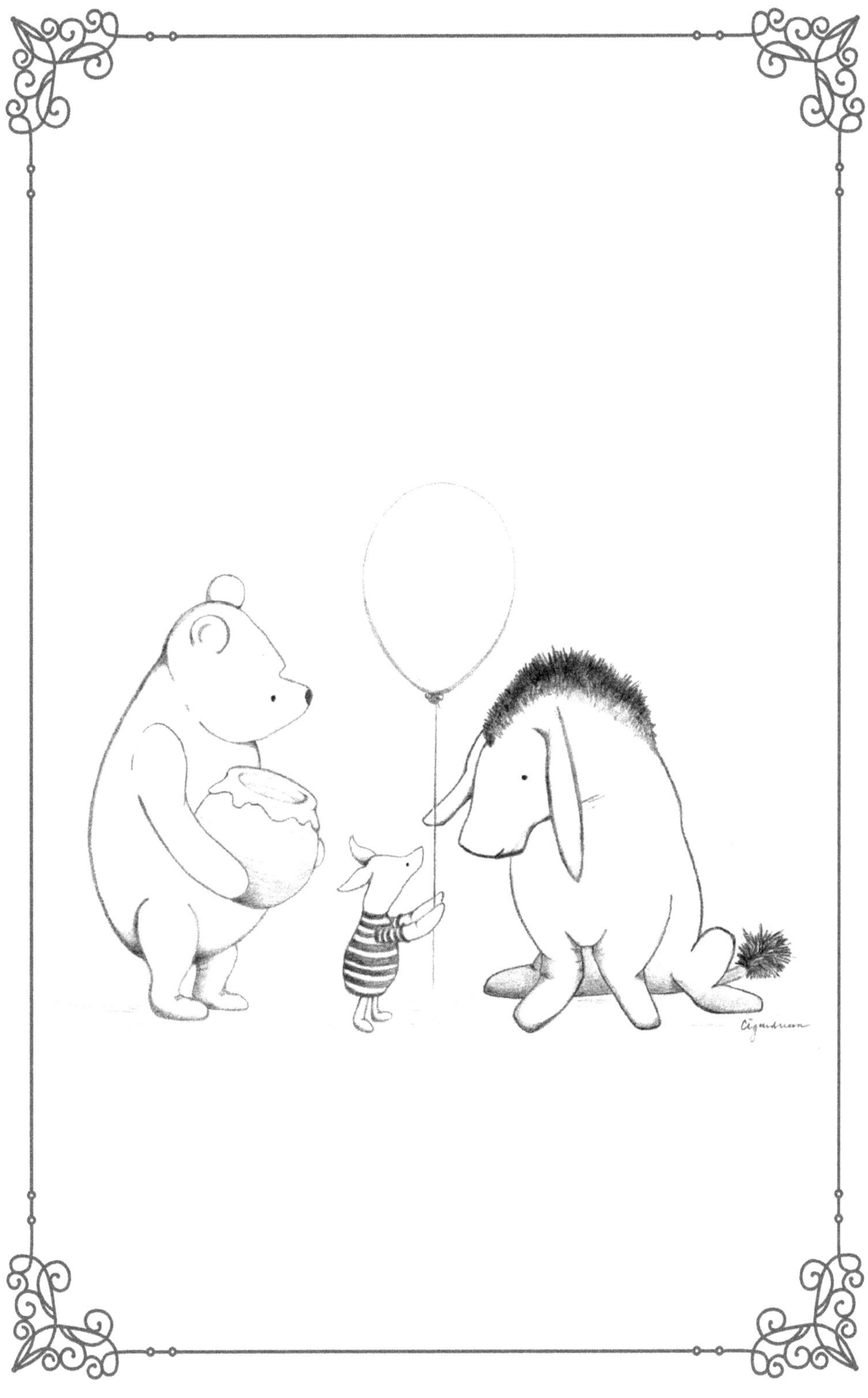

C is for Christopher Robin.

Pooh's best friend. He lovingly calls Pooh a
"Silly old bear".

**Call your best friend, or a family member to hear stories
of their life or success battling a disease or cancer.
Listen with your heart.**

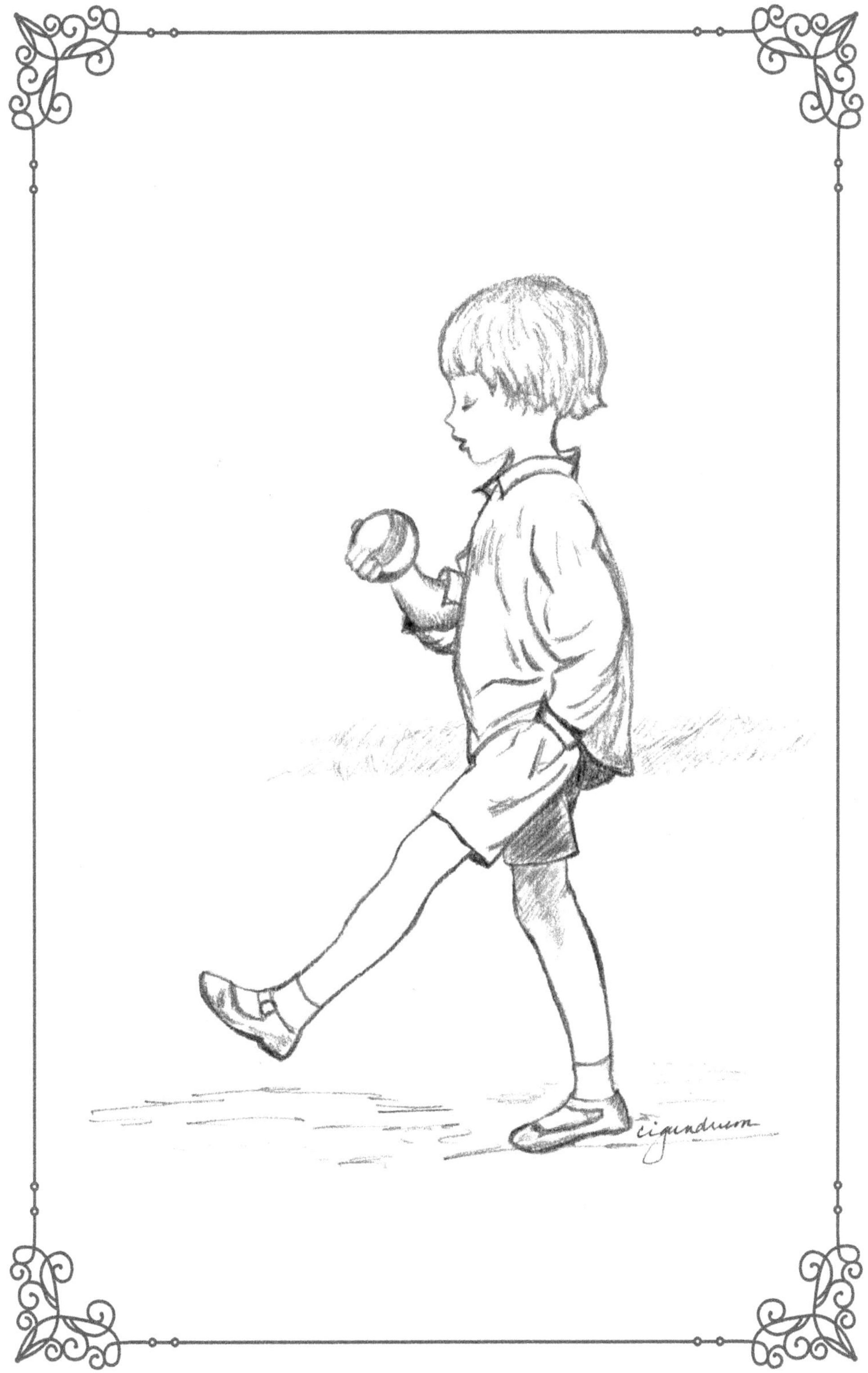

D is for a Difficult Day.

"Today was a Difficult Day," said Pooh.

There was a pause. "Do you want to talk about it?" asked Piglet. "No," said Pooh after a bit. "No, I don't think I do."

"That's okay," said Piglet, and he came and sat beside his friend. "What are you doing?" asked Pooh.

"Nothing, really," said Piglet. "Only, I know what Difficult Days are like. I quite often don't feel like talking about it on my Difficult Days either. "But goodness," continued Piglet,

"Difficult Days are so much easier when you know you've got someone there for you. And I'll always be here for you, Pooh."

And as Pooh sat there, working through in his head his Difficult Day, while the solid, reliable Piglet sat next to him quietly, swinging his little legs...he thought that his best friend had never been more right."

I am sending thoughts to you if you are having a Difficult Day today and hope you have your own Piglet to sit beside you or maybe you can cheer Eeyore up!

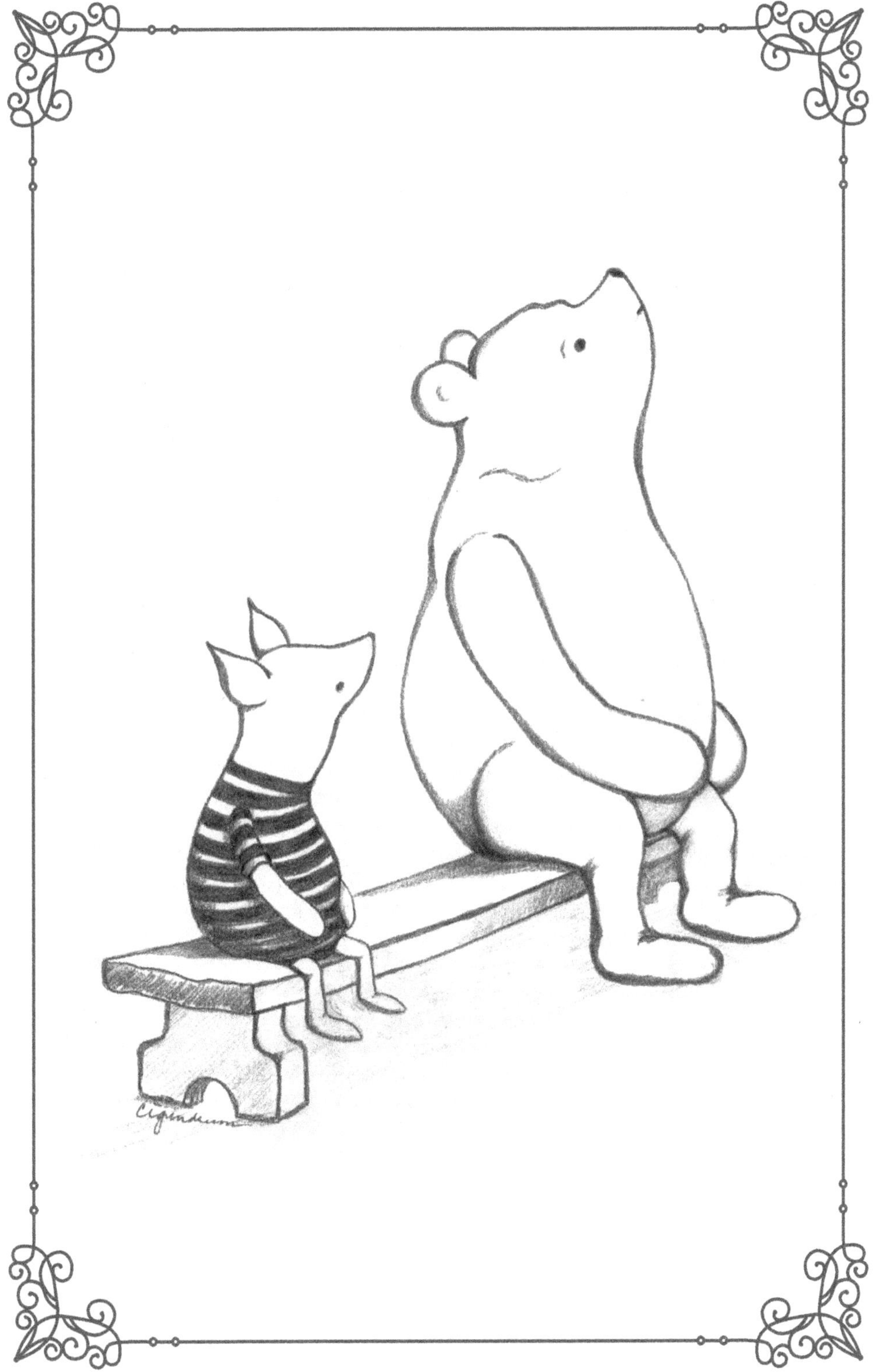

E is for Edward Bear.

That is Winnie-the-Pooh's real name!
Can you think of another character
that begins with the letter E?

Do you have a nickname? Many people do! I have a funny nickname from my dad and I have another nickname from kids at school. Write yours down here:

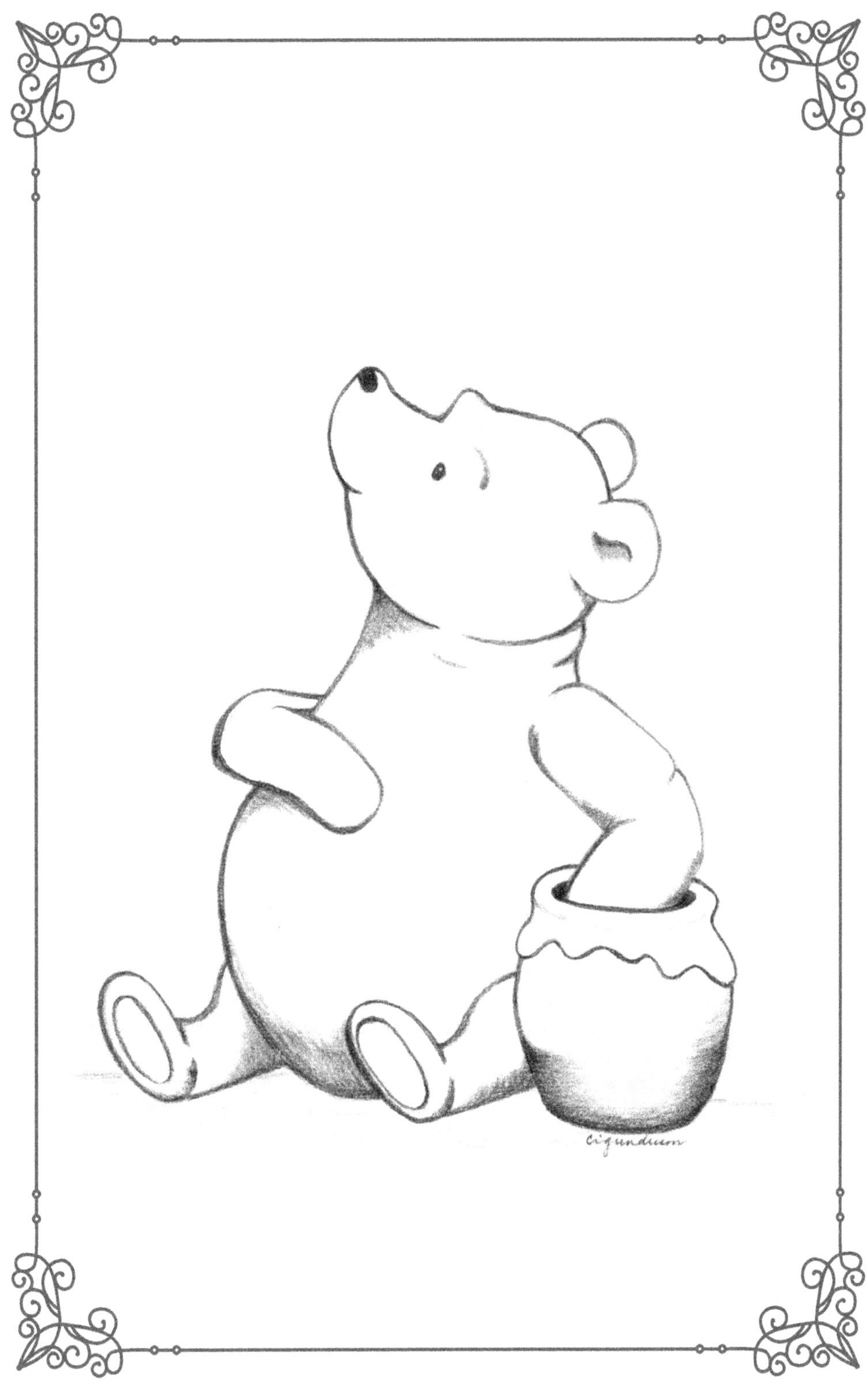

F is for Friendship

"A friend is one of the nicest things you can
 have and one of the best things you can be."
— Winnie

It's amazing to see your friends gather around you or think of
you. Don't be afraid to reach out to those you know. So often
friends and neighbors don't know how to approach cancer
patients for the first time. Be the first one to reach out.

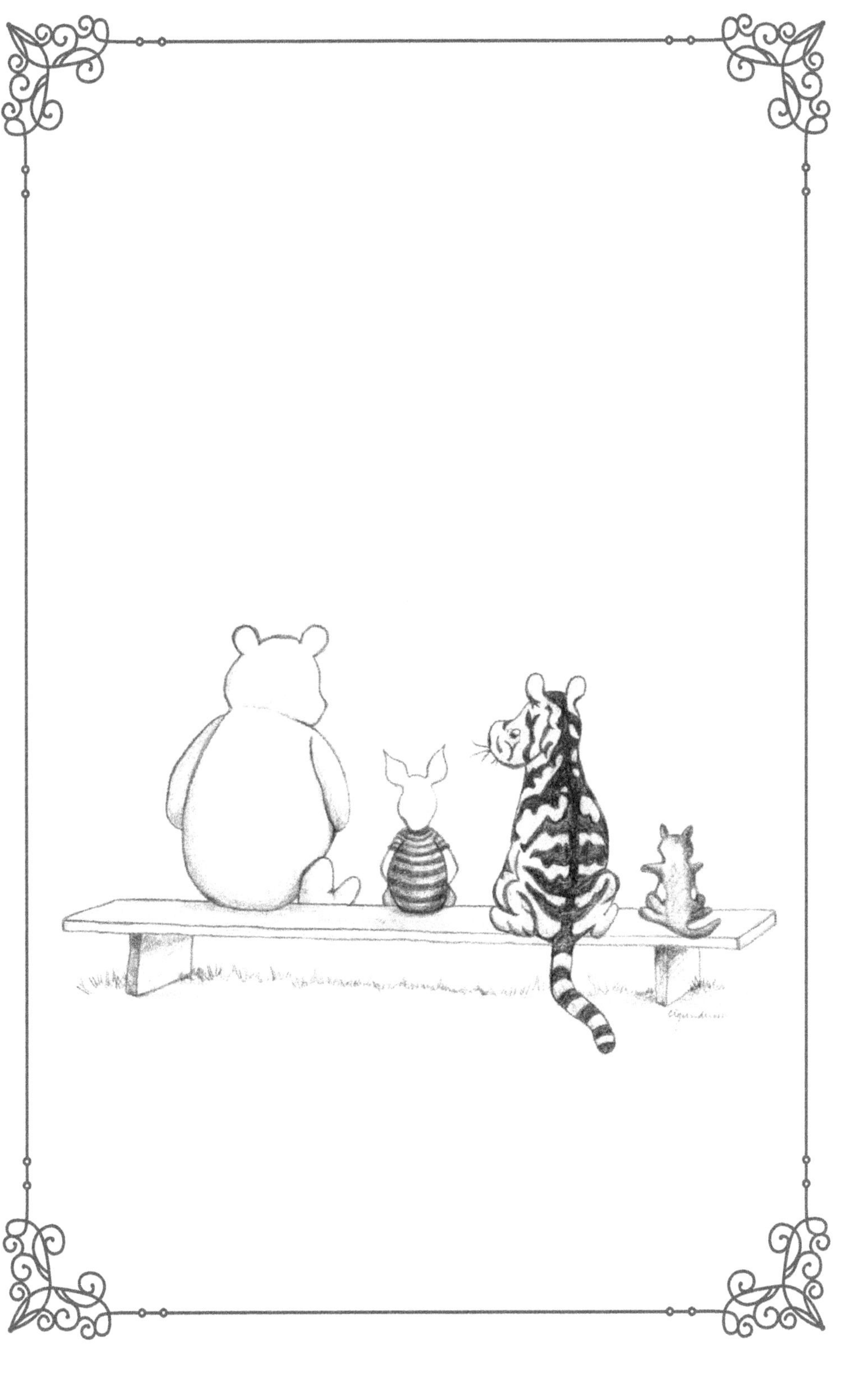

G is for Gratitude

"Piglet noticed that even though he had a very small heart, it could hold a rather large amount of gratitude."

Be sure to thank all your caregivers. The doctors, nurses, assistants, orderlies, techs, housekeepers, parents, relatives or friends. They are all helping you!

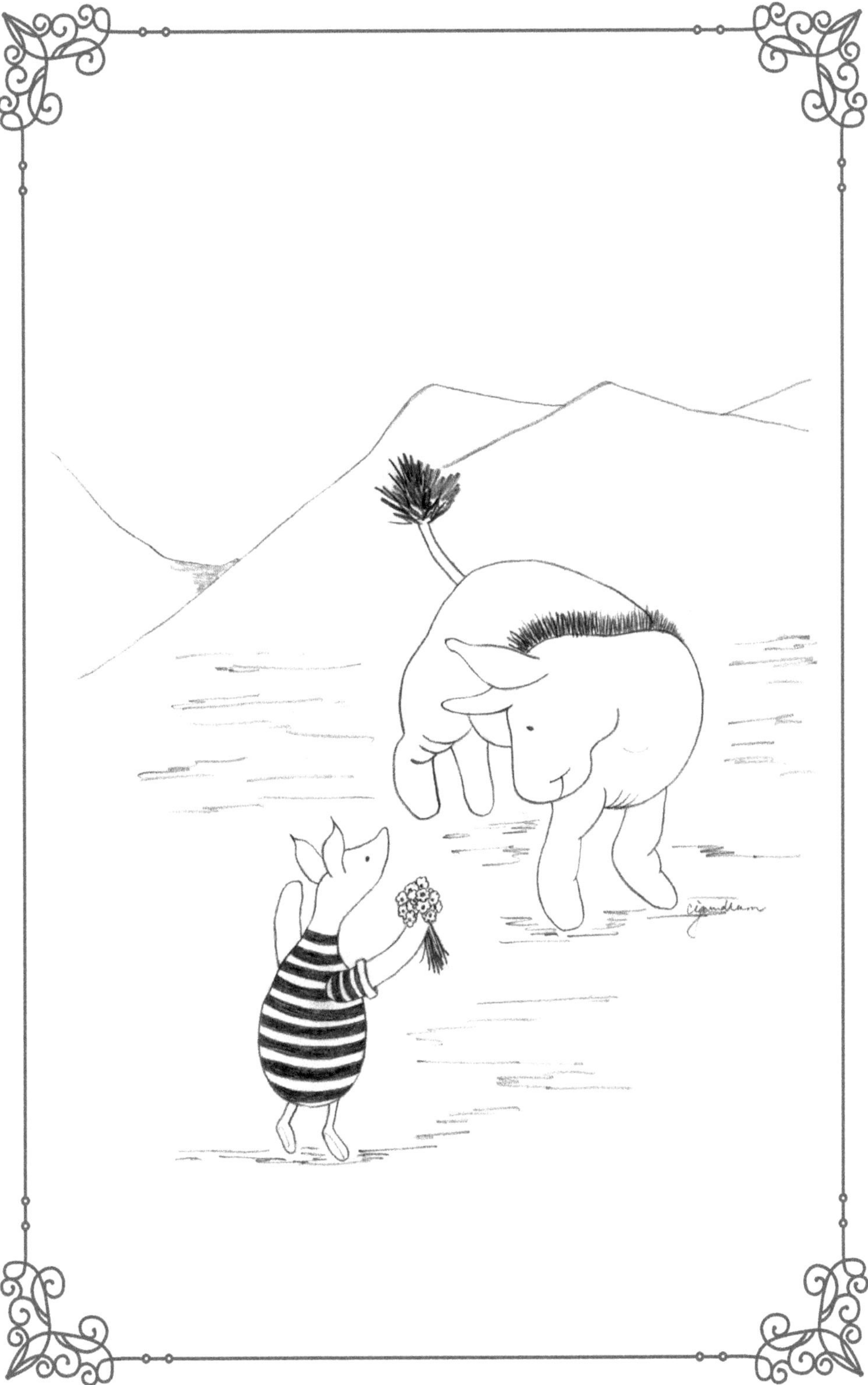

H is for Hug.

"A hug is always the right size,"

"Sometimes all you really need is someone to hug you tight and refuse to let you go until you feel better. You are very special." said Winnie.

Cancer isn't contagious. A hug from someone can be very healing. I love to give and receive hugs. Here's one especially for you!

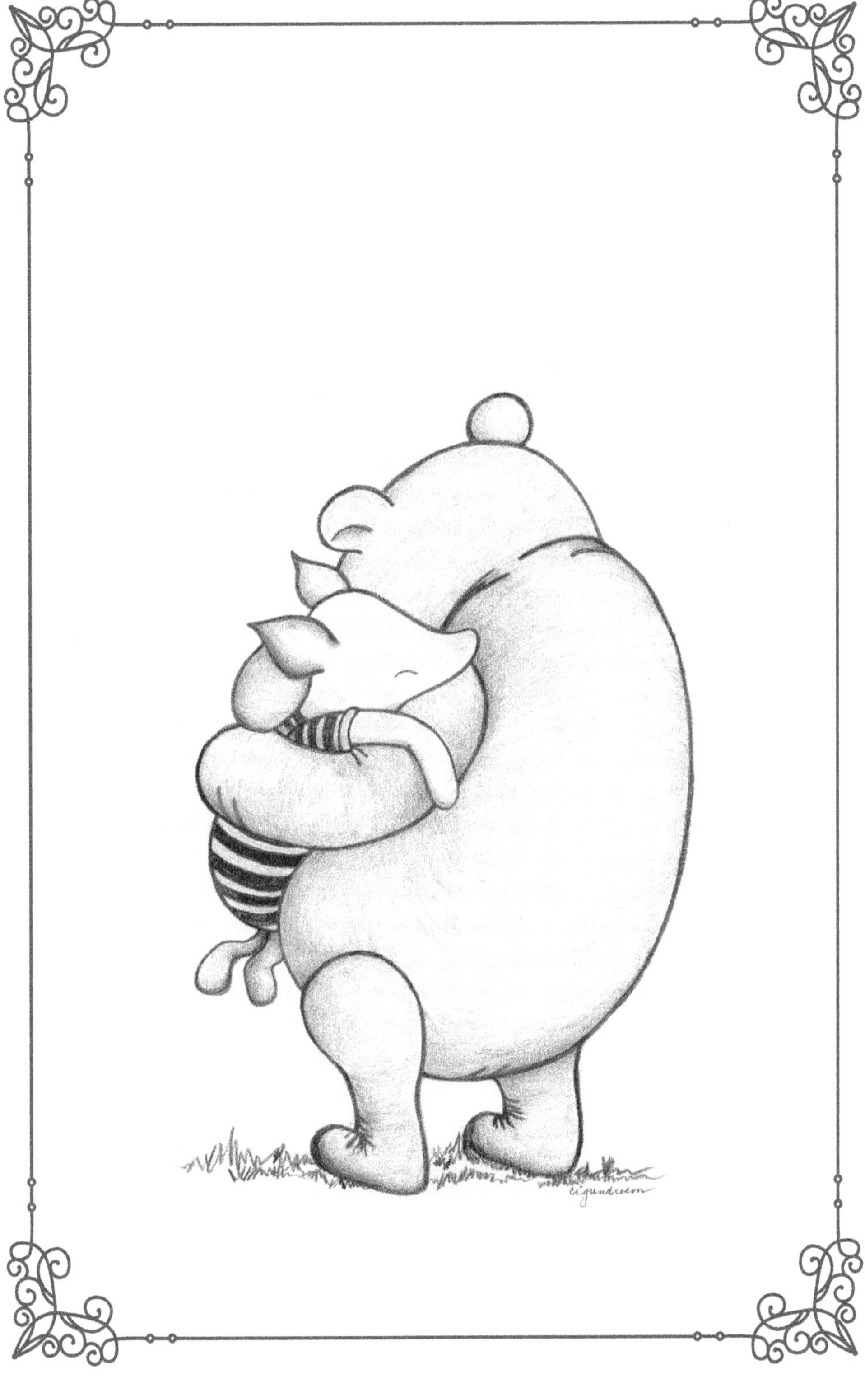

I is for I

"I always get to where I'm going by walking away from where I have been." — Winnie

I have been there. I am a Warrior. Being sick is a scary beginning to an adventure in life. Enjoy the things we forget to see when we are well. Be kind to yourself.

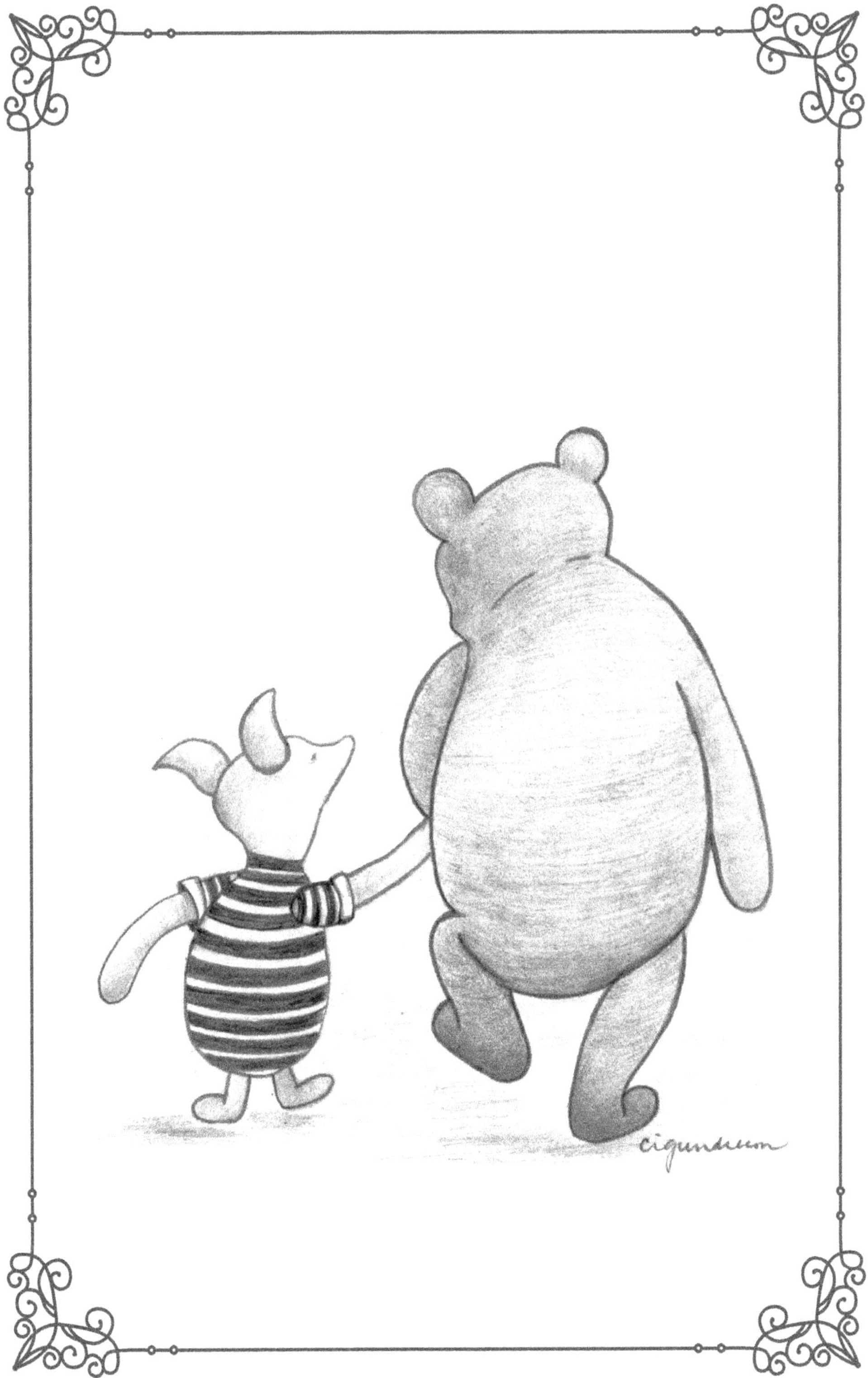

J is for Joey and Journal

A joey is a baby kangaroo. The joey in Winnie the Pooh's books is called Roo!

Roo loves to write in his journal but he is too little to print or write. But you can write or print in your journal, which is right after the letter Z! Take a look!

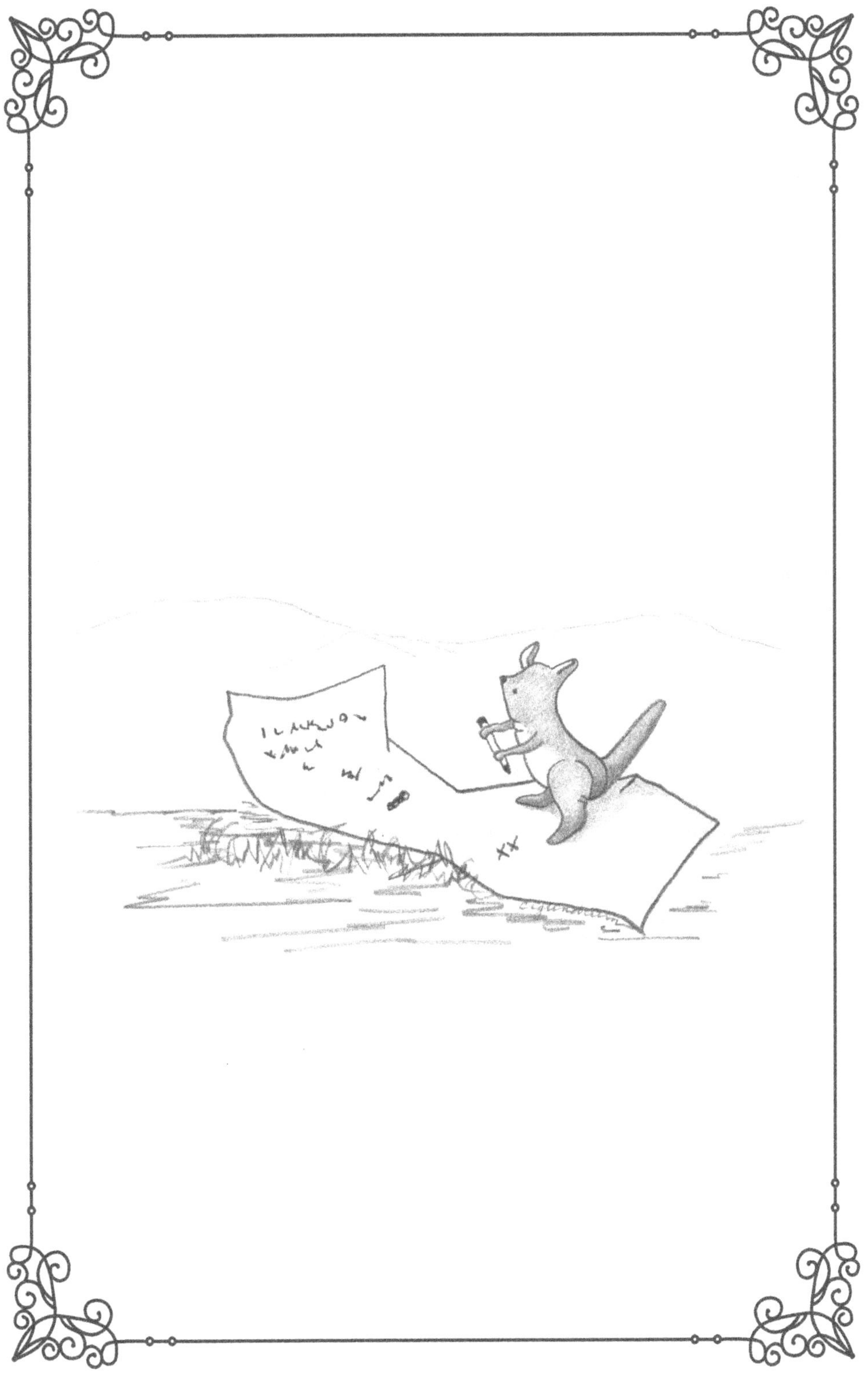

K is for Kanga.

This lovely doe (female kangaroo) takes very good care of her baby boy, Roo.

Let someone special be your Kanga and you be Roo.

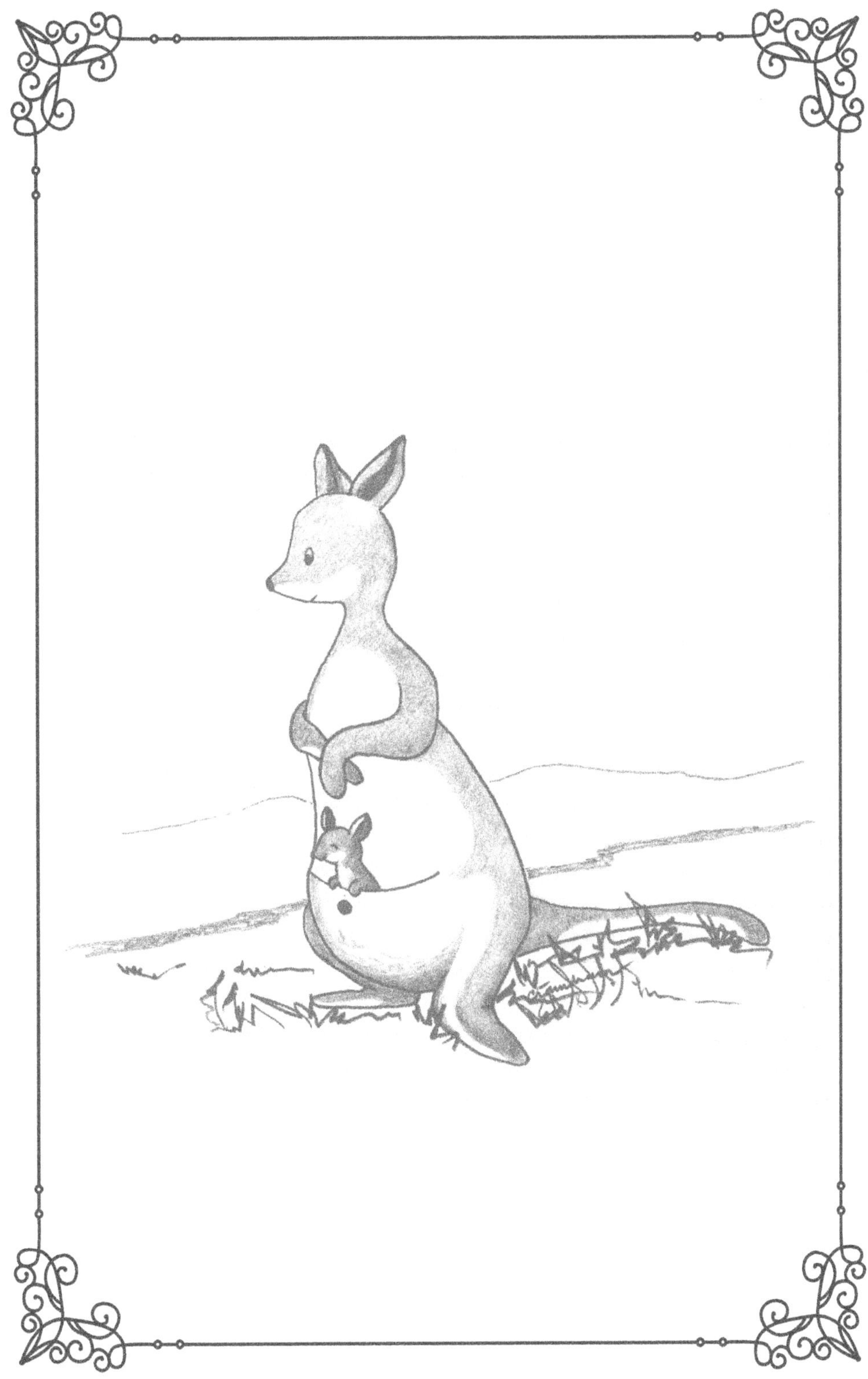

L is for Love.

"Some people care too much.
I think it's called love." — Winnie

"How do yo spell love?" asked Piglet.
"You don't spell it, you feel it." replied Pooh.

**It's amazing how many people love and care about you.
They love your strength, your attitude and just you.
You are amazing.**

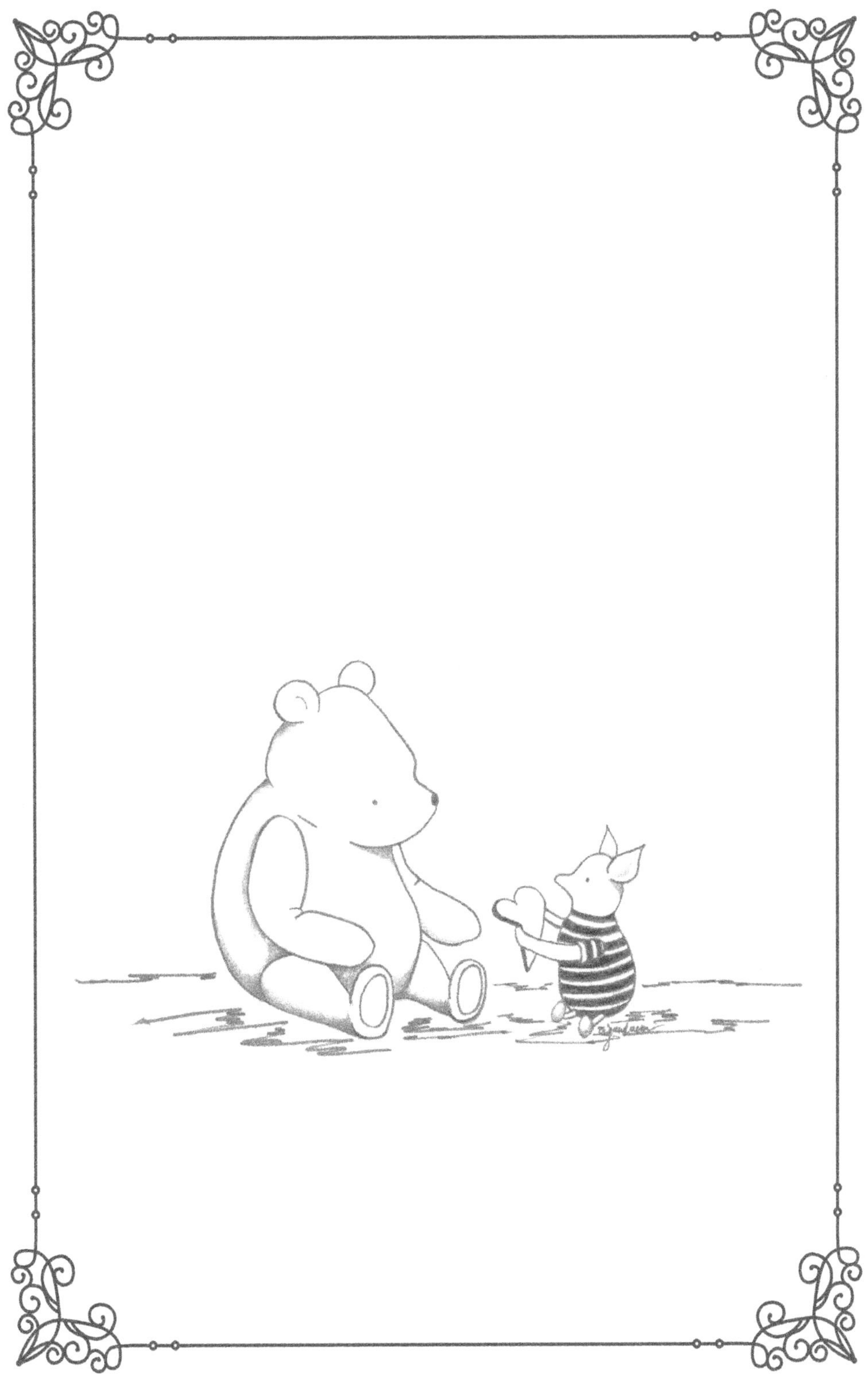

M is for Morning.

"When you wake up in the morning, Pooh,"
said Piglet, "what's the first thing you say
to yourself?"

"What's for breakfast?" said Pooh.
"What do you say, Piglet?"
"I say, I wonder what's going to
happen exciting to-day?" said Piglet.

Pooh nodded thoughtfully.
"It's the same thing," he said.

If your appetite is gone and nothing tastes like you remember, don't worry! It will come back. Try eating soft or canned fruit like mandarin oranges, watermelon, pineapple or high water fruits. Drink lots of fluids.

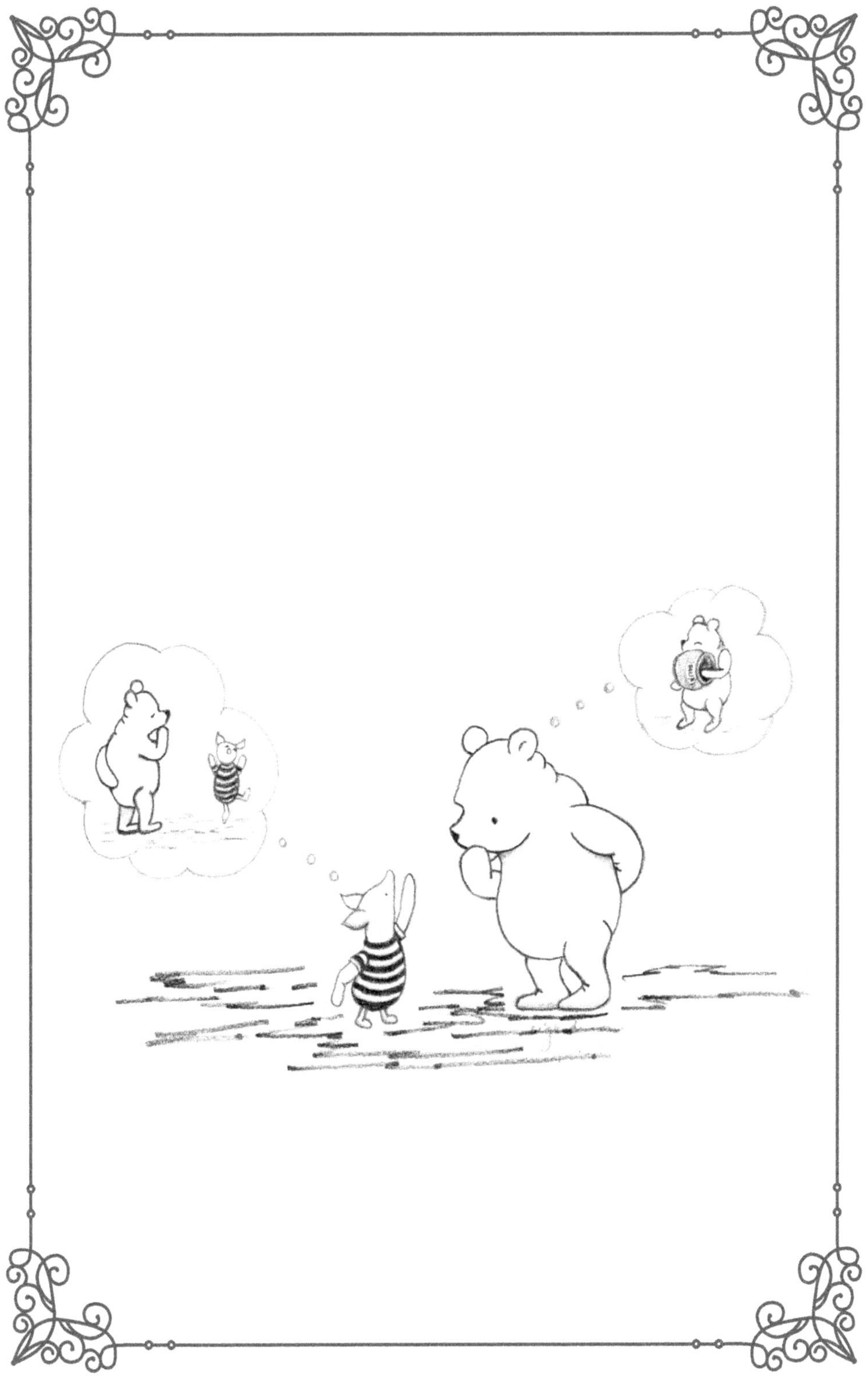

N is for Nothing.

"What I like doing best is nothing."
— Christopher Robin

"Don't underestimate the value of doing nothing."
— Winnie

"People say nothing is impossible...
but I do nothing everyday." — Winnie

If you do nothing every day, that's ok! Your job is to get better. Let your medical team do the work. Let your friends and neighbors lend a hand if you need help with anything!

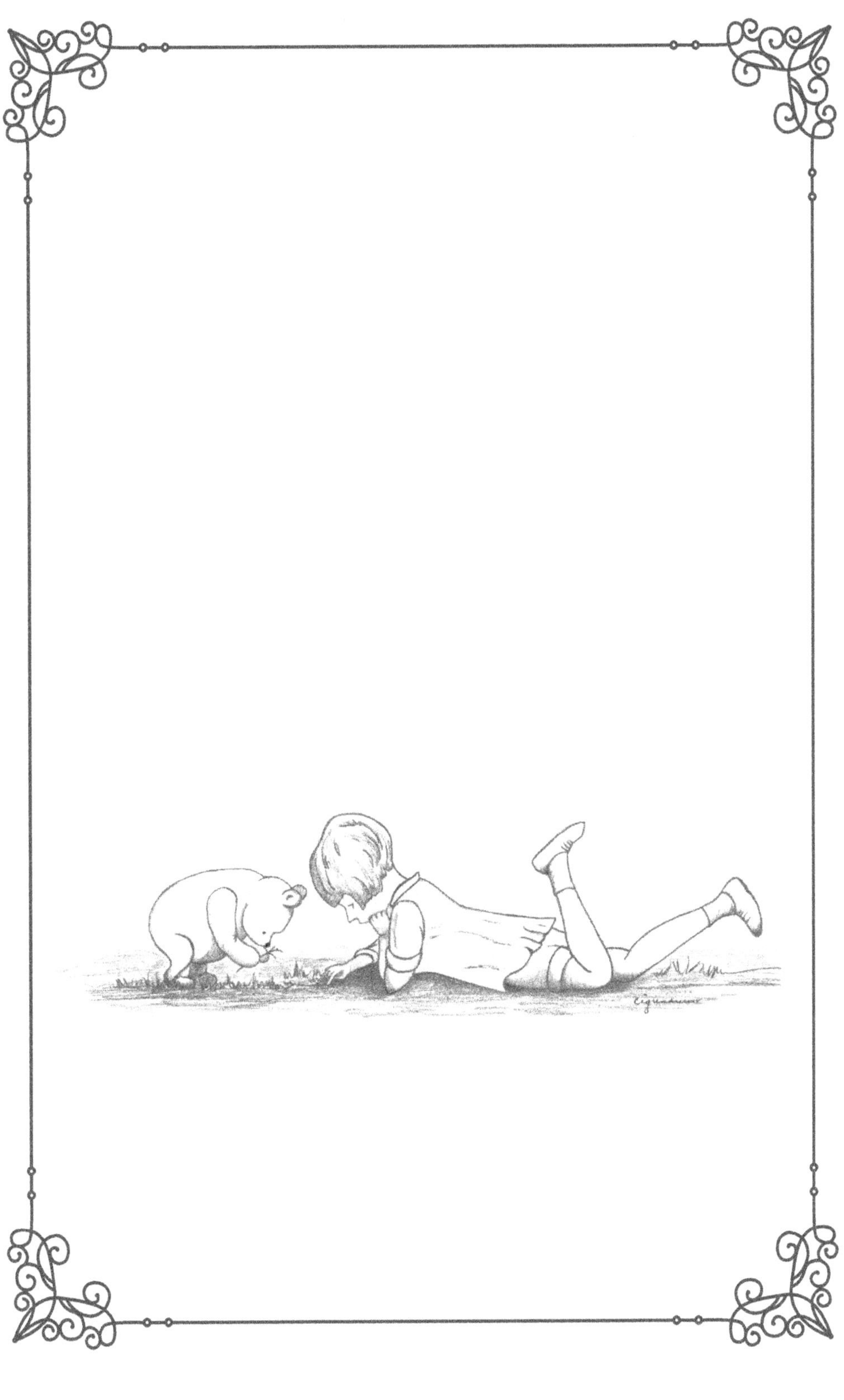

O is for Ok.

"It's ok to not be ok. Some days
are just harder than others," said Eeyore.

Isn't that the truth! It's ok to not get up in the morning.
It's ok to have as many naps as you want. It's ok to use
a walker if your balance is off. Be kind to yourself.

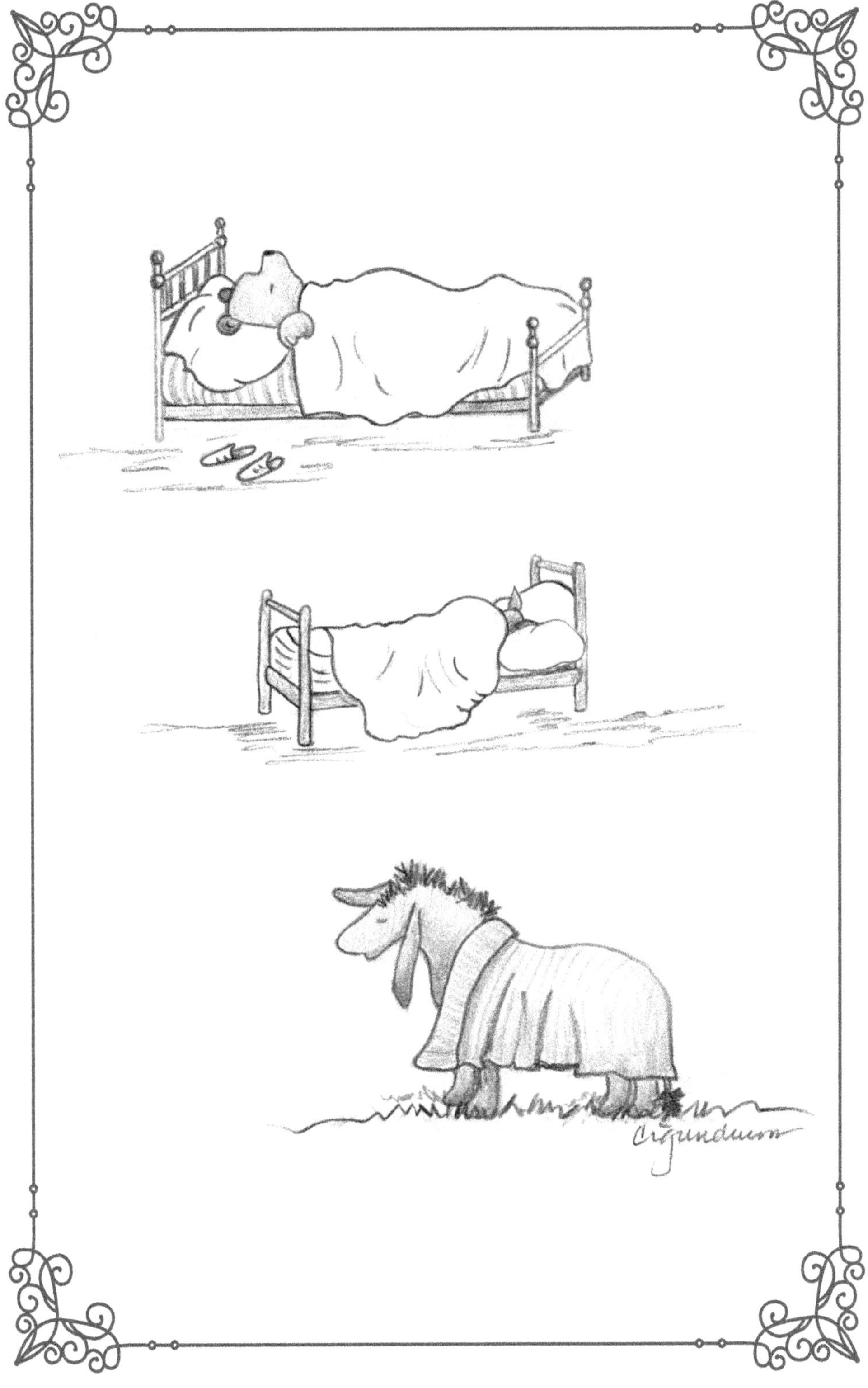

P is for Piglet.

"The things that make me different are
the things that make me, me." said Piglet.

**You are the only you. First and foremost you are a treasure.
Show your strength and get up when you fall. If you can't get
up by yourself take a helping hand from someone but get up.
You are a Warrior and I love that about you.**

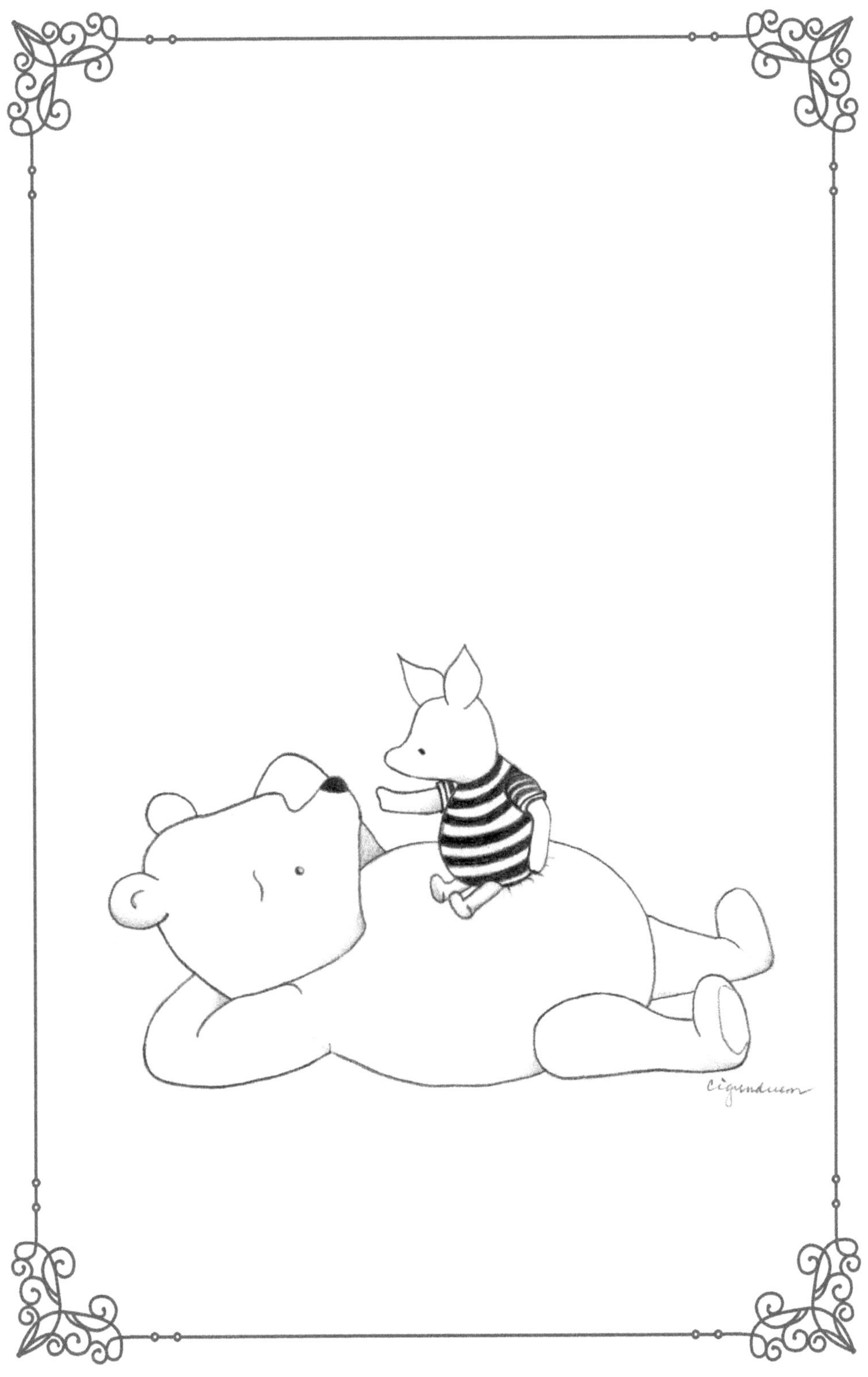

Q is for quiet thinking.

"If the person you are talking to doesn't appear
to be listening, be patient. It may simply be that
he has a small piece of fluff in his ear."

"I wonder how many wishes a star can give."
— Winnie

**Enjoy the quiet. Busy places can be very noisy. Find a place
where there are no noises that bother you. It might be inside
or outside. Put some fluff in your ears!**

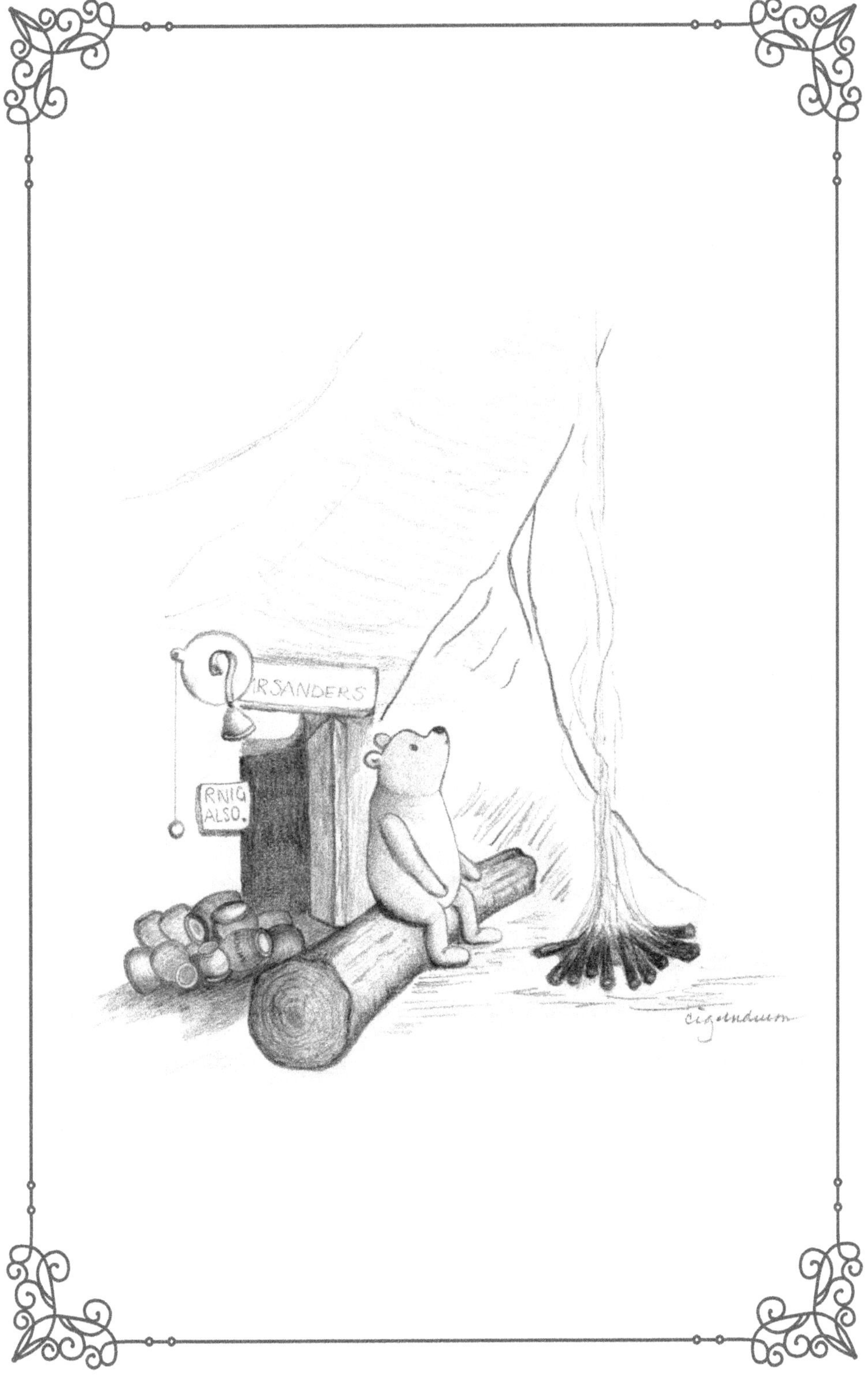
RSANDERS
RNIG
ALSO.

R is for Room.

"Sometimes the smallest things take up the most ROOM in your heart." — Winnie

What takes up the most room in your heart? I hope it's love.

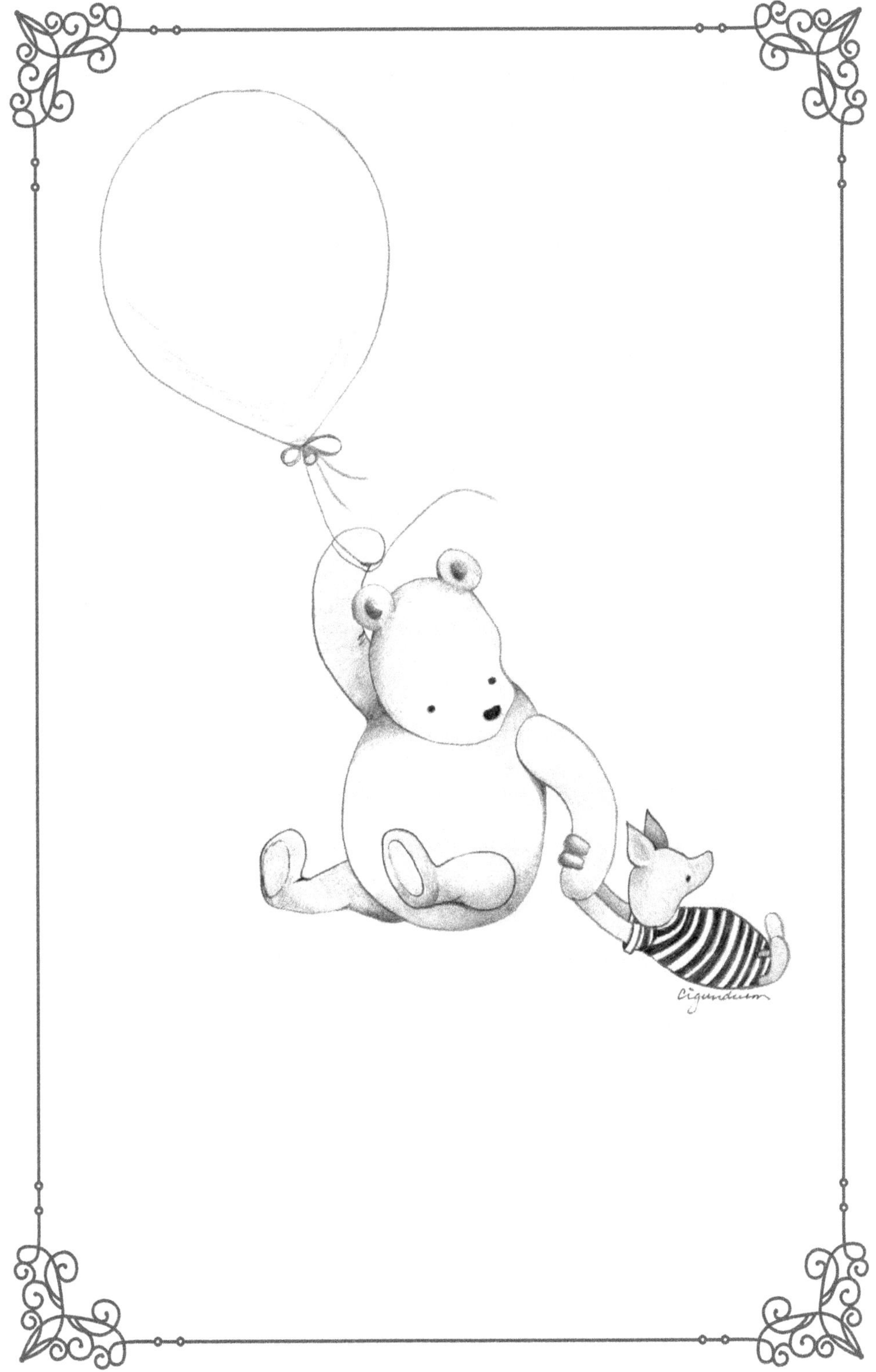

S is for Strength.

"You're braver than you believe, stronger than you seem and smarter than you think," said Christopher Robin

Play a game of solitaire or work on a puzzle. Try a few gentle exercises while sitting or holding onto something for support. Keep your body and mind active.

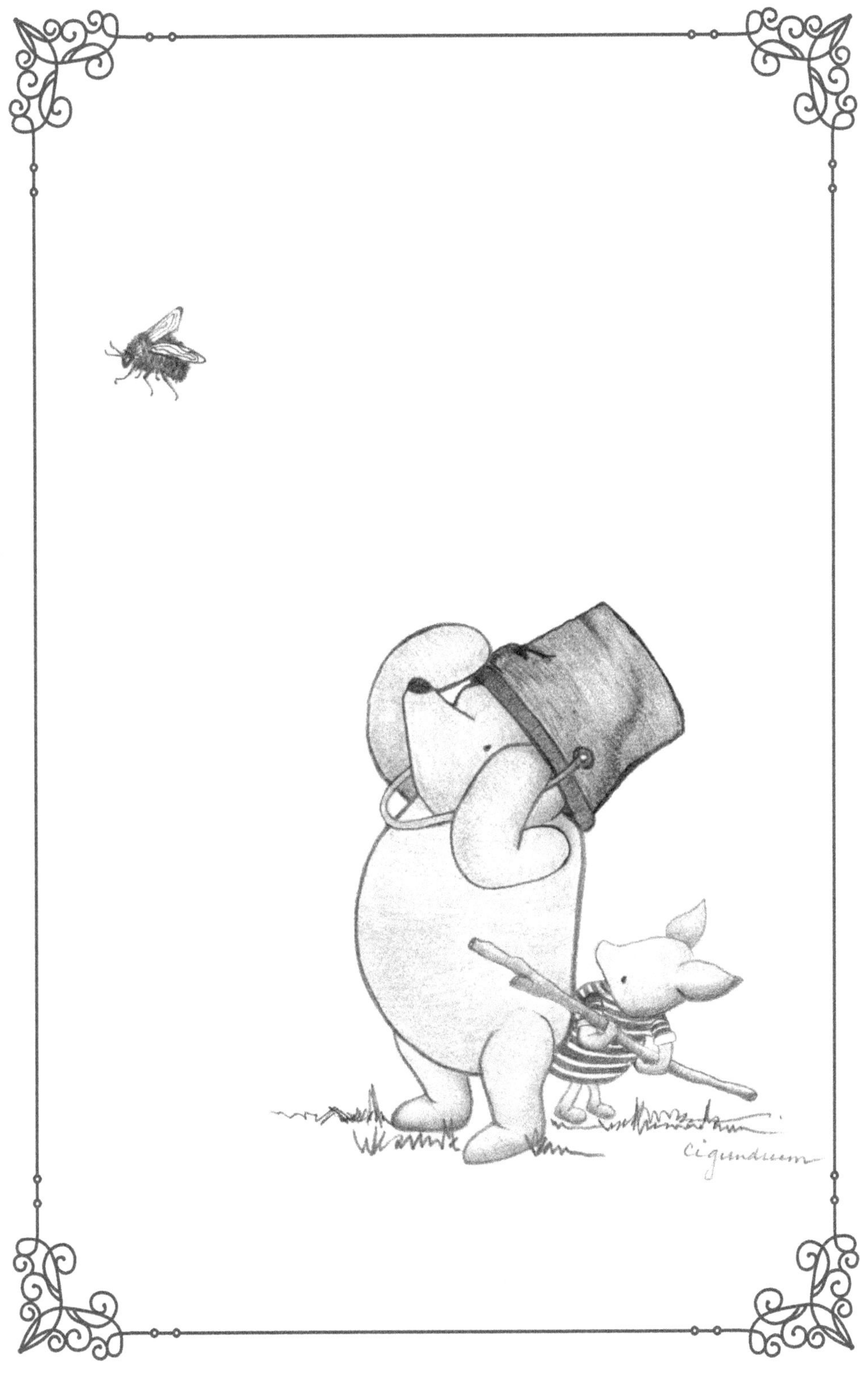

T is for Together.

"If there ever comes a day when we can't
be together, keep me in your heart,
I'll stay there forever," said Winnie the Pooh

Many days you can't be together with your family or friends because of distance or work. Find a way to connect. It is hard when you live alone or are in the hospital. If you're at home, I hope you have a pet (great listener) or have joined a support group. If you're in the hospital, ask if they have a therapy dog that will visit you. If not, give your special teddy or stuffy a hug.

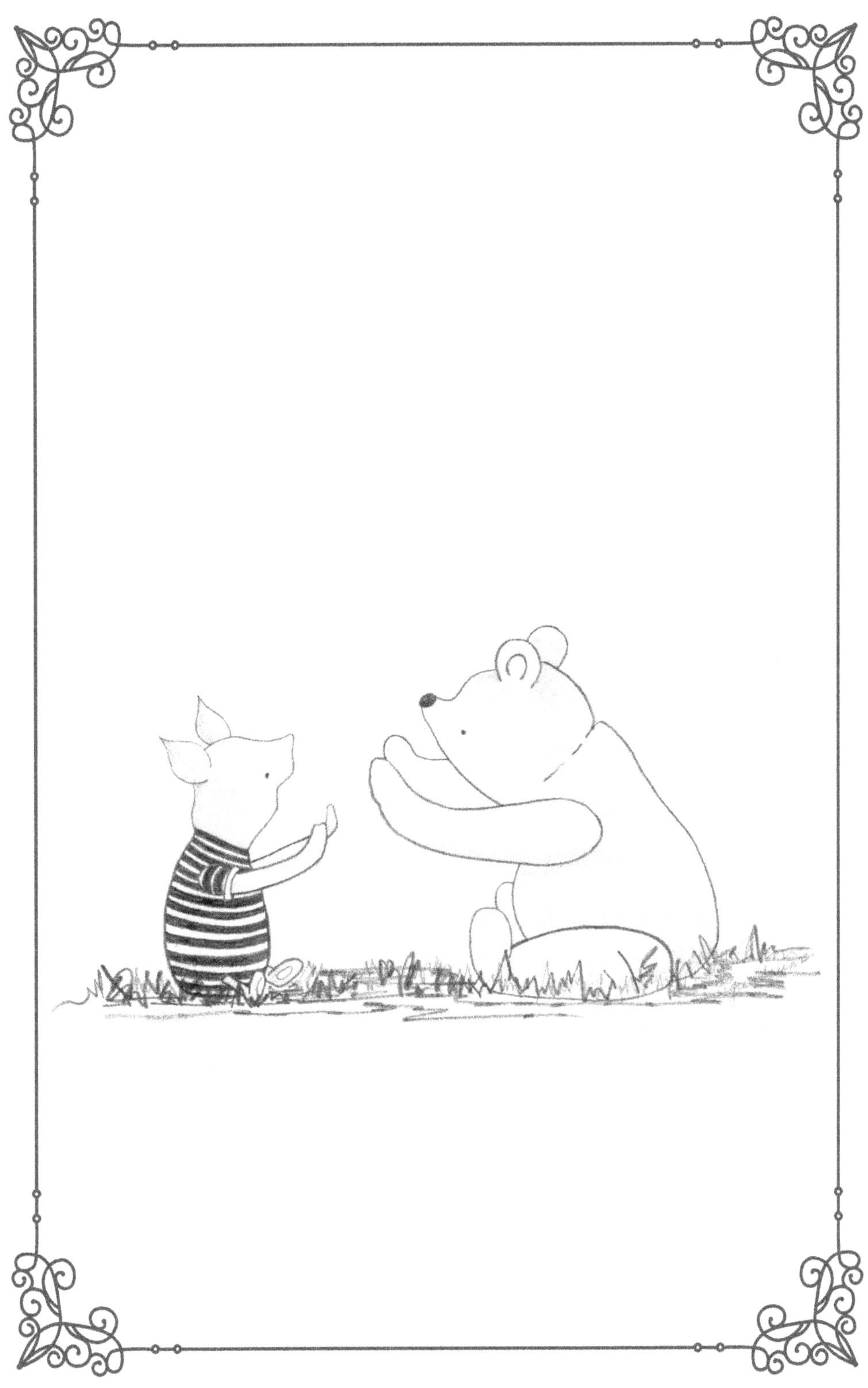

U is for Upset.

"I was so upset, I forgot to be happy," said Eeyore.

Some days you will feel like this. Give yourself time to reflect on happy memories or happy thoughts. Read or watch something that makes you happy.

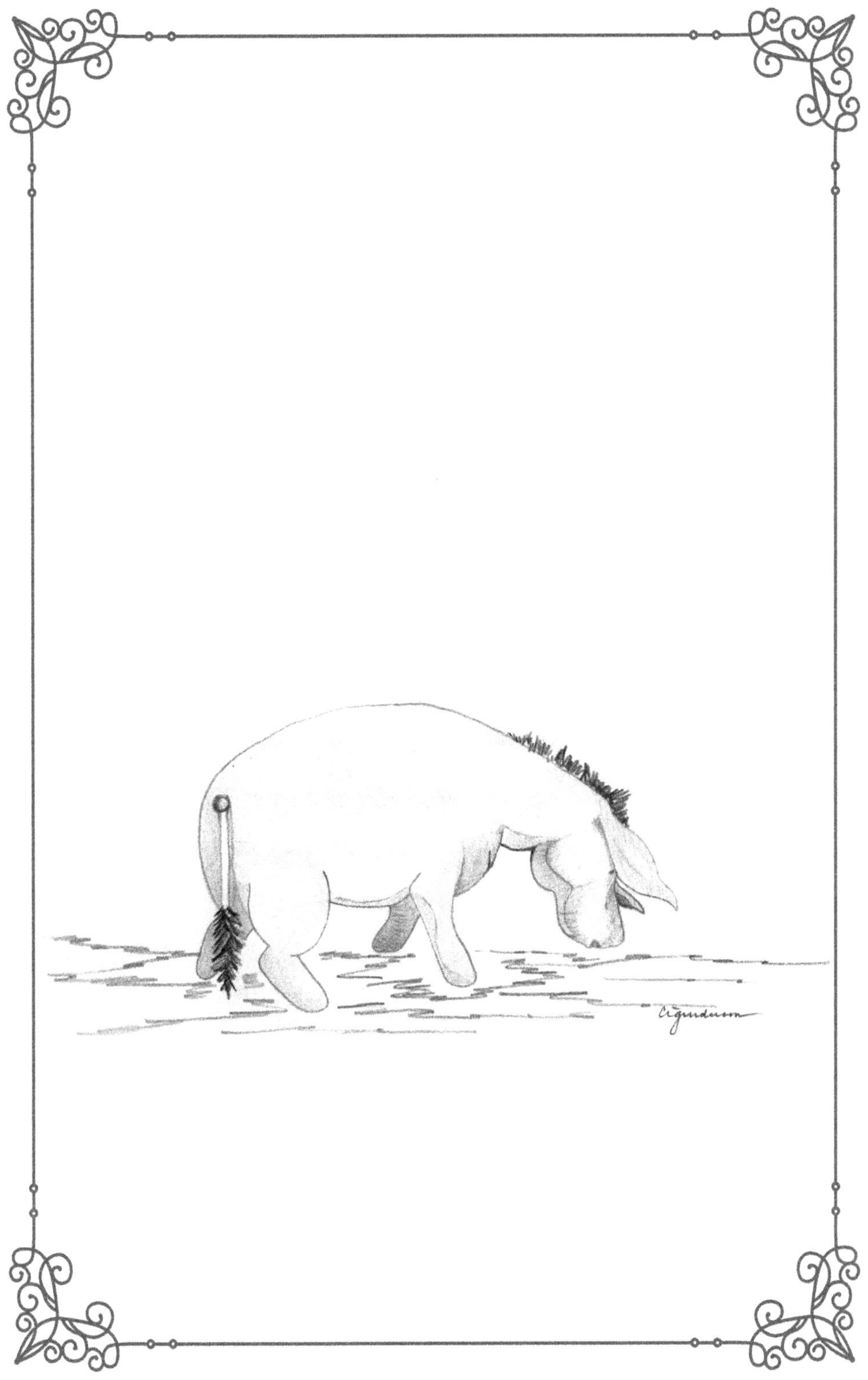

V is for VOICE.

Winnie the Pooh & Rabbit: "Hello, Rabbit,"
he said, "Is that you?"

"Let's pretend it isn't," said Rabbit, "and see
what happens."

Piglet: "It is hard to be brave when you're only
Very Small Animal."

Eeyore: "They're funny things, accidents.
You never have them until you're having them."

Roo: "Look at me jumping!"

**Pretend you are these characters. Say their words in a VOICE
that matches the character!**

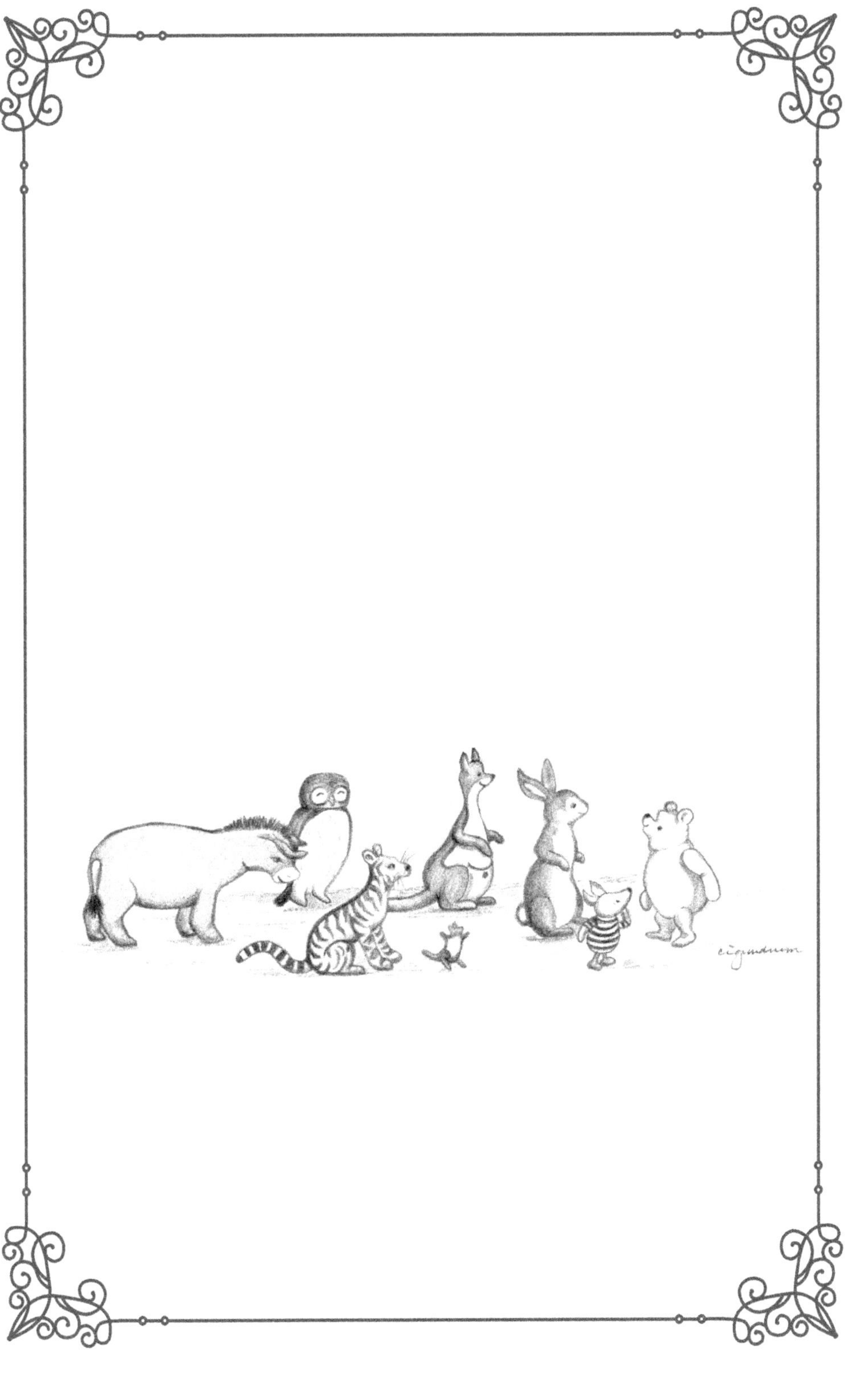

W is for Wobbly.

WOL is an OWL. He thinks he's a wise old owl and signs his letters WOL, which he thinks spells OWL.

"My spelling is WOBBLY. It's good spelling but it Wobbles, and the letters get in the wrong places."
— Winnie the Pooh

You may find that you can't print or write properly after medications. Don't fret about it! Your printing and writing will return eventually. Using technology is a great way to communicate.

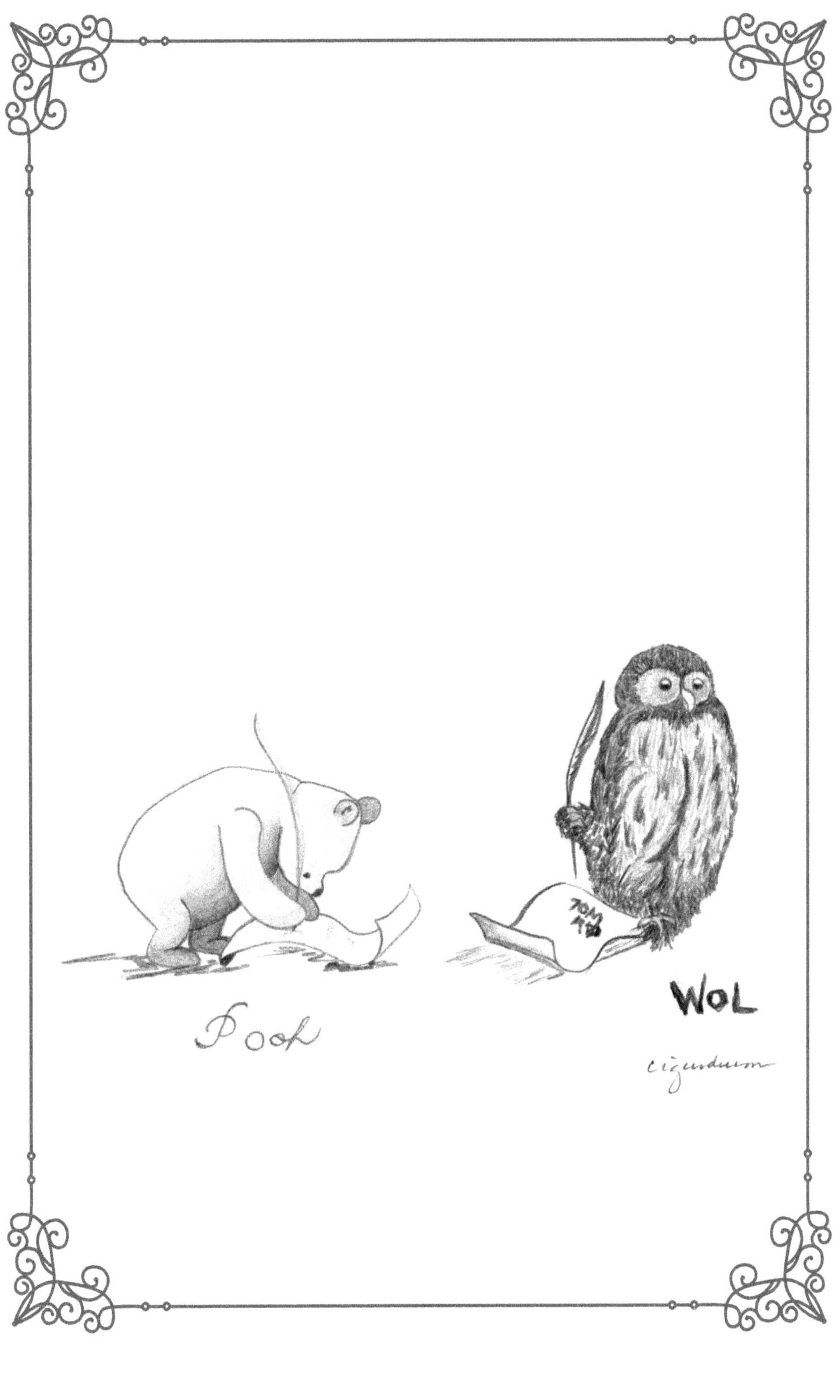
Pooh
WOL

X is for X-RAY.

We all know what this one is! But what is the difference between an X-ray, CT (CAT) Scan, MRI and PT (PET) Scan?

X-ray: An X-ray is a quick, painless test that produces images of the structures inside your body. Bone and metal show up as white, air in your lungs shows up as black and fat and muscle show up as shades of gray. X- ray is an abbreviation for X Radiation. The "X" means "unknown". The scientist who discovered the X-ray didn't know what to call it, so he named it "X"!

CT or CAT: A CT or CAT scan is a combination of X-rays and a computer to create pictures of your organs, bones, and other tissues. It shows more detail than a regular X-ray. It is a quick and painless test. CT is an abbreviation for Computerized Tomography.

MRI: An MRI scanner uses strong magnetic fields, magnetic field gradients, and radio waves to generate images of the organs in the body. An MRI does not use radiation. It is a painless procedure. MRI is an abbreviation for Resonance Imaging.

PET: A PET scan is an imaging test that can reveal the metabolic function of your tissues and organs. The PET scan uses a radioactive drug called a tracer to show both normal and abnormal metabolic activity. PET is an abbreviation for Positron Emission Tomography.

If Winnie wasn't stuffed with fluff, this is what he thinks his x-ray would look like.

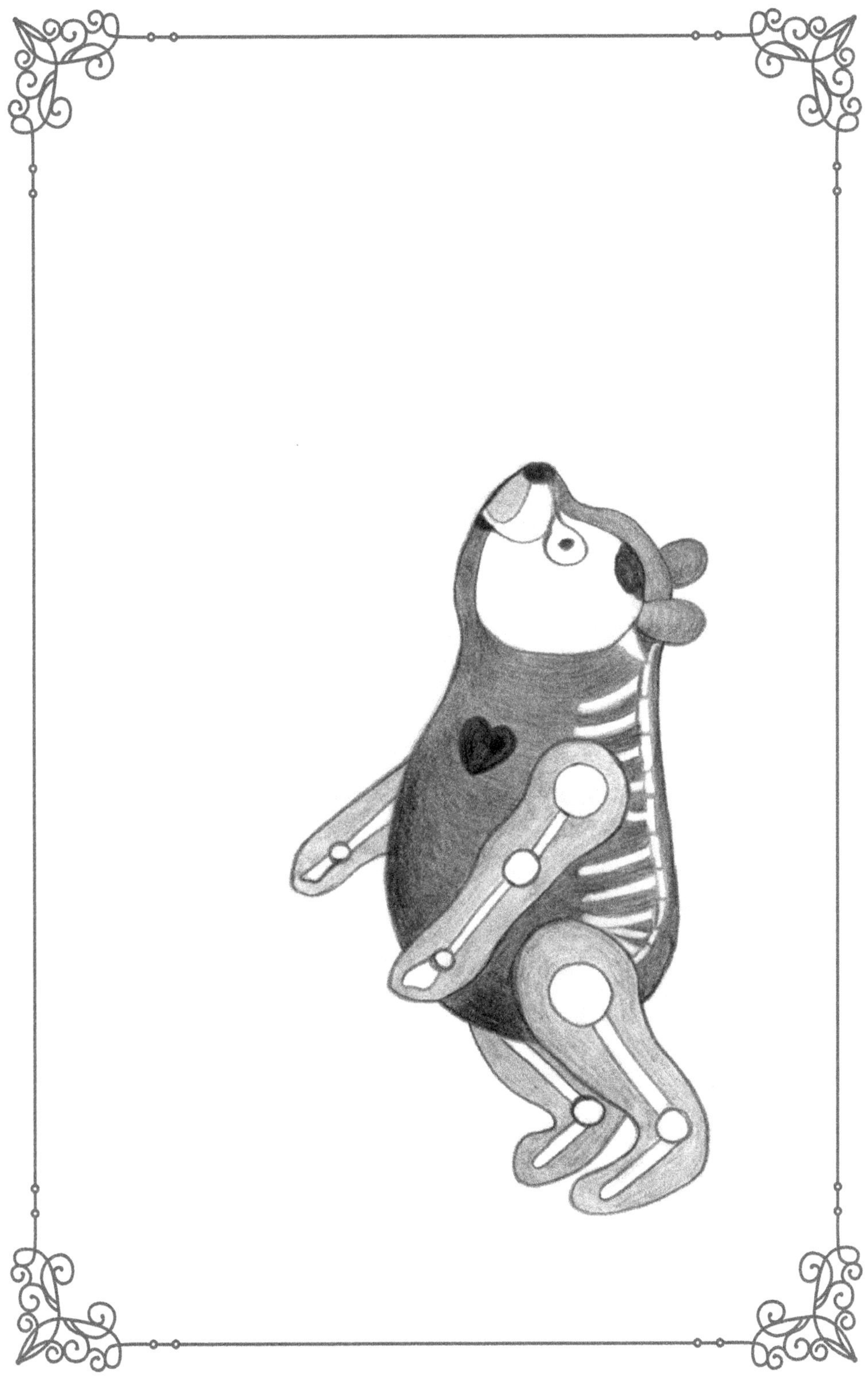

Y is for You.

"I love you simply because you're YOU."
— Winnie

"Any day spent with YOU is my Favorite Day.
So today is my New Favorite Day." — Winnie

"If you live to be 100, I hope to live to be 100
 minus 1 day, so I never have to live without YOU."
— Winnie

**YOU are what this book is all about. YOU are a Warrior.
YOU are a fighter. We need YOU!**

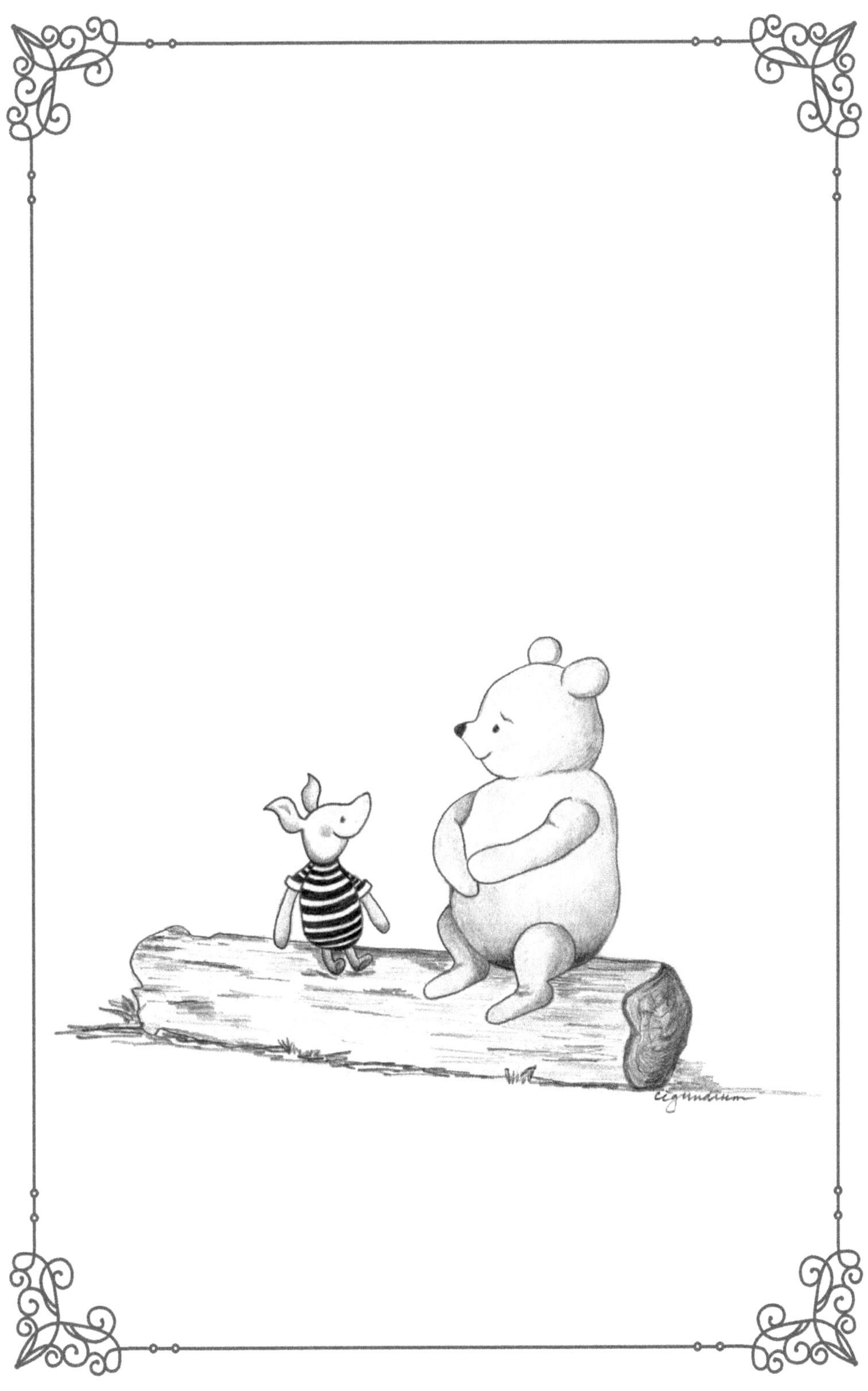

Z is for Zee or Zed.

Did you know that the letter Z is pronounced ZED in The United Kingdom, Canada, and other Commonwealth Countries?

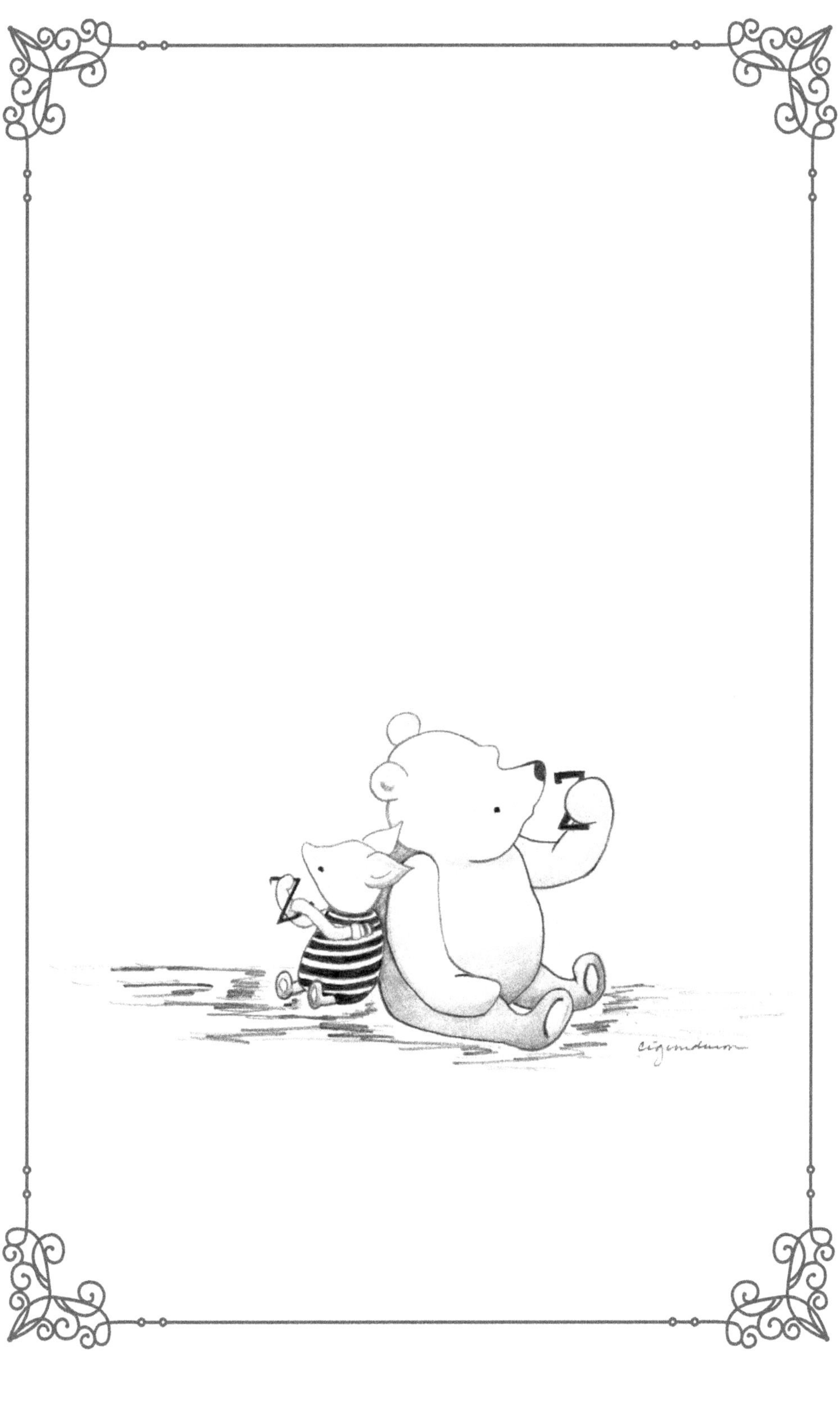

My Journal

Here's a place to write your thoughts,
designs and doodles.

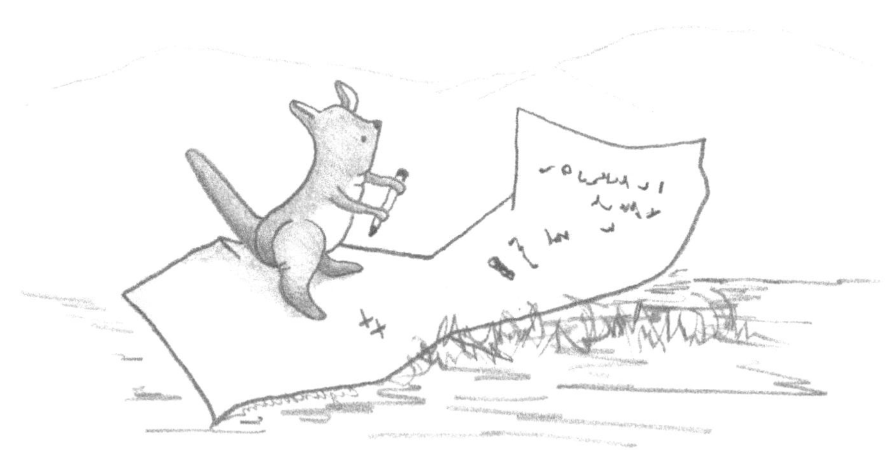

A is for...

B is for...

C is for...

D is for...

E is for...

F is for...

G is for...

H is for...

I is for...

J is for...

K is for...
L is for...

M is for...

N is for...

O is for...

P is for...

Q is for...

R is for...

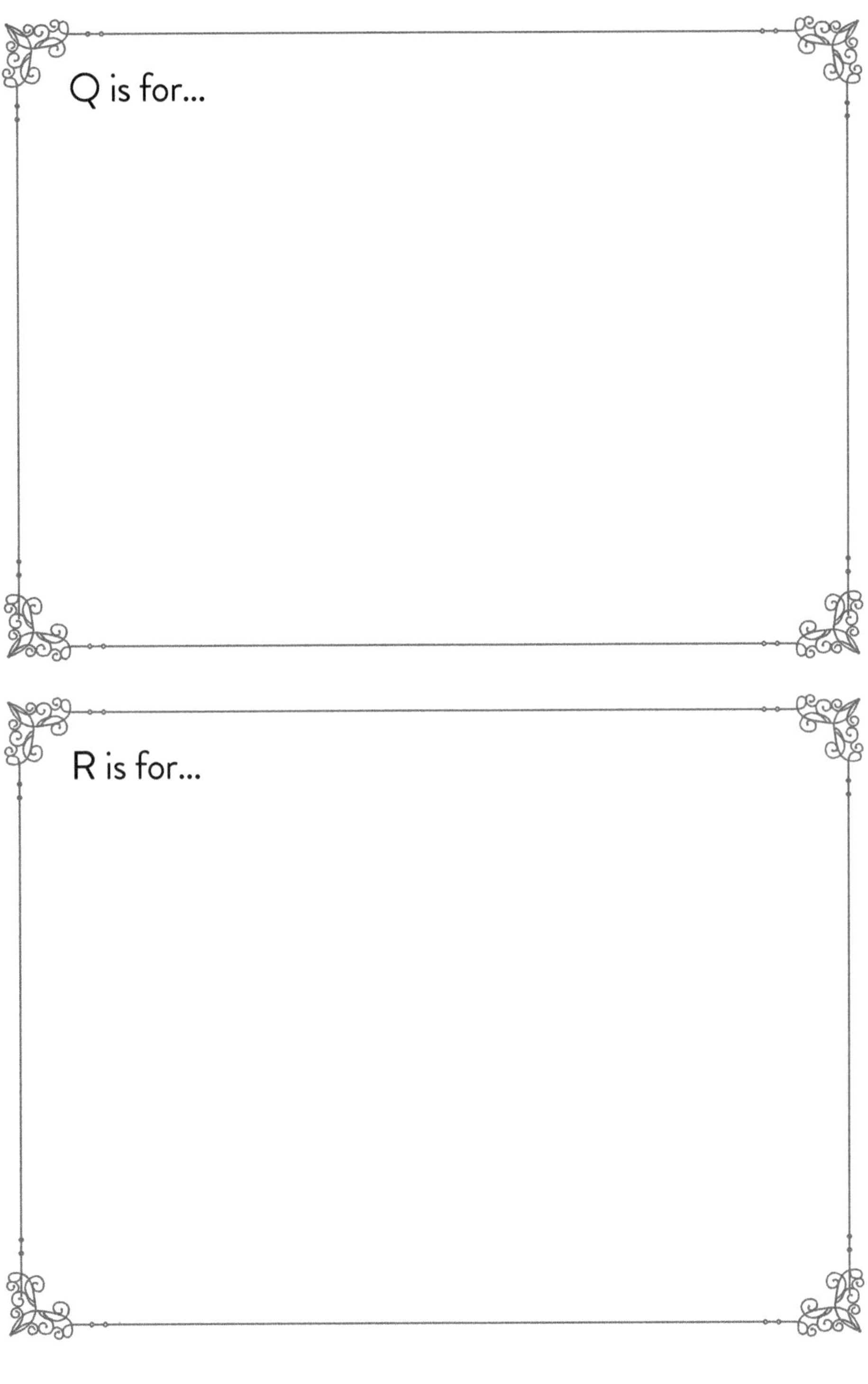

S is for...

T is for...

U is for...

V is for...

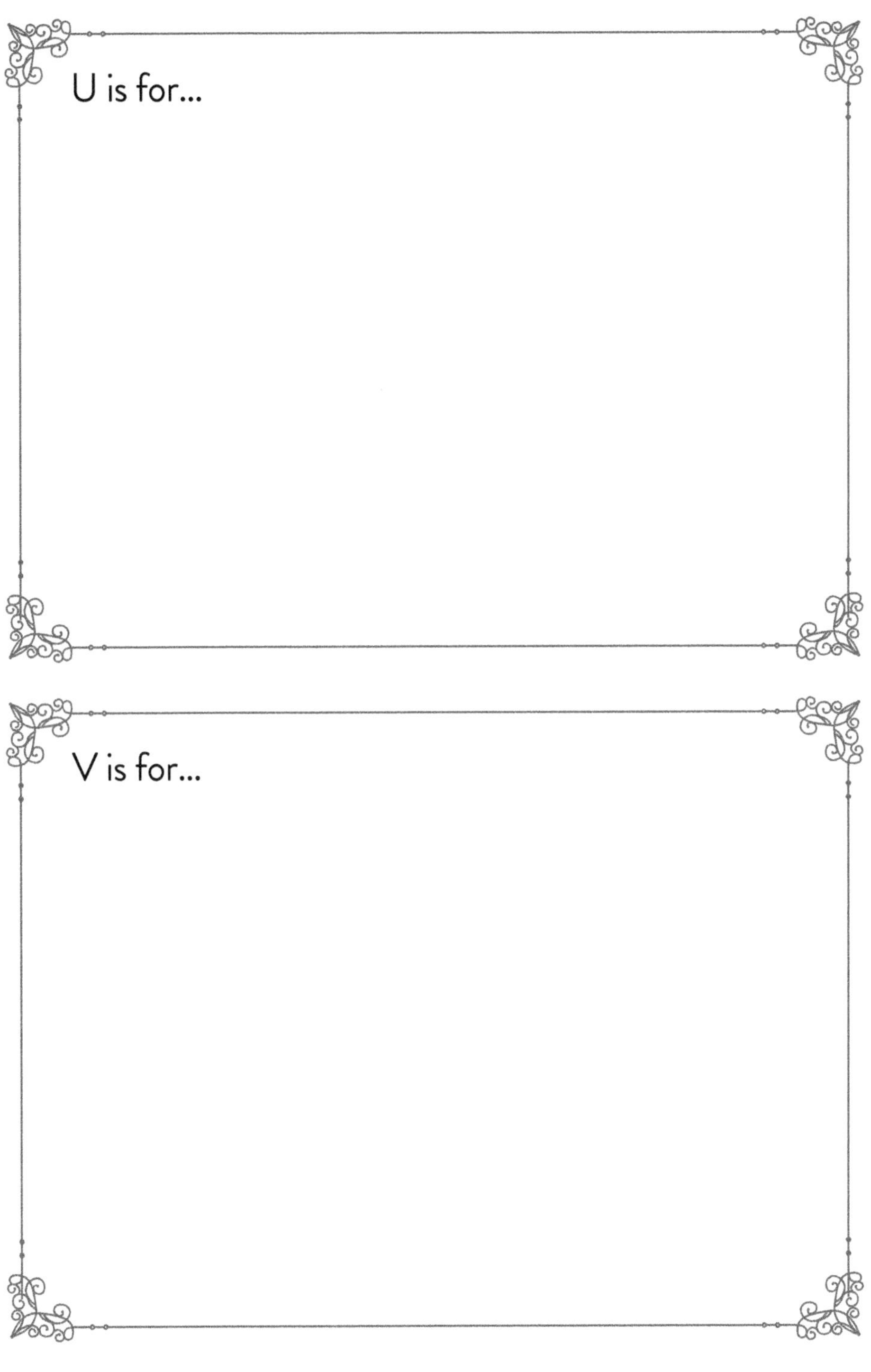

W is for...

X is for...

Y is for...

Z is for...

Winnie the Pooh or Winnie-the-Pooh was created by British author A.A. Milne in the 1920s. Milne based the characters on his son, Christopher Robin, his stuffed animals—Winnie the Pooh and friends Piglet, Eeyore, Kanga, Roo and Tigger—
who all lived in their country home in England's Ashdown Forest.

My drawings are inspired by Mr. E.H. Shepard. He was
a British illustrator and cartoonist, best known for his
illustrations in A.A. Milne's "Winnie-the-Pooh" books.
He created the iconic images of Winnie-the-Pooh, Piglet,
Tigger, and other characters that have become synonymous
with the classic children's tales. Shepard's imaginative and
whimsical illustrations have made a lasting impact on the
world of children's literature and continue to be loved by
generations of fans.

Carolyn Gundrum taught kids to love reading. She was a
Library/Media Specialist in Kelowna, B.C., Canada; Holland,
Michigan; Fishers, Indiana and Las Vegas, Nevada.
She moved to Norman, Oklahoma to be near her sister but one
day felt Ill. It turned out to be Non-Hodgkin Lymphoma! After a
year of chemo, radiation and many scans, she is now NED (No
Evidence of Disease).

This is my first book. My inspiration came from my kids
and friends. I hope this book inspires you.

When I was going through my treatments, one thing kept
popping up… cancer patients need inspiration and good
thoughts to keep going!

If you liked this book, I would love for you to leave a review on
Amazon.com or wherever you purchase finer books.

Email me at gundrumpc@gmail.com to tell me your thoughts.
I promise I will write back to you.

Thank you!

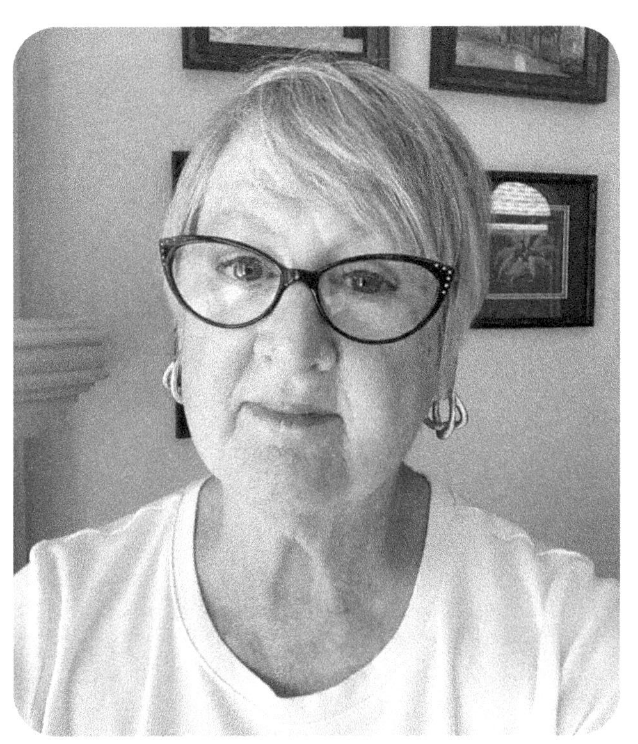